T0191454

RESEARCH AND STUDY SKILLS FOR VETERINARY NURSES

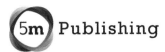 Publishing

RESEARCH AND STUDY SKILLS FOR VETERINARY NURSES

Jane Davidson

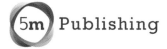

5m Publishing

First published 2019

Reprinted 2021

Copyright © Jane Davidson 2019

Published by
5M Publishing Ltd,
Benchmark House,
8 Smithy Wood Drive,
Sheffield, S35 1QN, UK
Tel: +44 (0) 1234 81 81 80
www.5mpublishing.com

A catalogue record for this book is available from the British Library

ISBN 9781789180138

Book layout by
Keystroke, Neville Lodge, Tettenhall, Wolverhampton

Printed by Replika Press Pvt Ltd, India

Photos and illustrations by the author unless otherwise indicated

Chapter opening photos from Adobe Stock: Ch 1 © Vitaliy;
Ch 2 © Helder Almeida; 3 © fantom_rd; Ch 4 © karmad;
Ch 5 © paylessimages; Ch 6 © Светлана Валуйская; Ch 7 © Eva;
Ch 8 © Pictures news; Ch 9 © Stephanie Zieber

Online resources available from https://www.5mbooks.com/study-skills

Contents

For Hollie, my soul mate, my daemon, my constant shadow and to all the Hollies who need a vet nurse to save them.

About the author

Jane RVN was a late convert to vet nursing after taking a degree in history and spending some time selling wine. However, it was the career she always wanted and she has never looked back.

She qualified as an RVN in the UK via the NVQ route and then took her learning further, completing the Post Graduate Diploma in Professional and Clinical Veterinary Nursing.

Educating the vet nurse community has always been a passion. Jane gained her assessor/clinical coach status and is also an internal verifier. To support her teaching, she has completed her Diploma in Teaching in the Lifelong Learning Sector, a Level 3 coaching and mentoring course and a Pg Cert in Clinical Education and gained her Fellowship of the Higher Education Academy (FHEA). She has taught the theory and practical aspects of the Level 3 Diploma and on a BSc in veterinary nursing.

In practice, she enjoys anaesthesia and theatre duties and has a passion for the geriatric patients and end of life care.

Jane uses social media to communicate and educate via @JaneRVN and the award winning #PlanetRVN

She believes every vet nurse student can achieve academic success if they use the right tools to help them.

Vet nurse education – for everyone, everywhere

Hello everyone it's Jane RVN, and welcome to this comprehensive guide to succeeding in your vet nurse training and beyond.

I'm a UK based registered veterinary nurse and I have been for over 15 years, arriving quite late to the industry after being waylaid by a history degree and the wine industry. But I found my calling and during my career I have worked in charity and private practices covering day and emergency shifts. I have also been a clinical coach, an internal verifier, OSCE examiner and lecturer. If qualifications are your thing then I have:

- MA in History from Glasgow University
- NVQ3 in Vet Nursing
- GradDipVN in Practical and Clinical Vet Nursing from Royal Veterinary College
- Diploma to Teach in the Lifelong Learning Sector – DTLLS
- Internal Quality Assurance – IQA
- Post Graduate Certificate Clinical Education from Edinburgh University
- Fellowship of the Higher Education Academy.

In practice and in college I have seen the struggles facing vet nursing students, particularly the limited resources and time available to students to improve their academic skills. Improving academic skills might seem a world away from cleaning a kennel but it is only with academic skills to understand the clinical skills we use that a vet nurse can improve throughout their career.

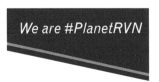

This book is for everyone training as a vet nurse or vet tech across the globe. The vet nurse community

We are #PlanetRVN

is now connected worldwide, and best practice and new innovations are shared easily. Social media helps us greatly and I use #PlanetRVN to share ideas, thoughts and research. It's a popular # and won an RCVS Innovation Award in 2017. Share your ideas and plans for studying, revision and research on Twitter, Instagram and Facebook with #PlanetRVN or @JaneRVN.

The joy of social media is bringing us all together. While in each country our numbers are small, across the world we are a big community. We all have a passion to improve the health and welfare of our patients. Our patients range from cats and dogs to birds, fish and all manner of wildlife. What we have in common is a desire to learn more to improve their lives.

> *I have found vet nurses in all corners of the globe helping where they are needed.*

We all carry on learning once we're qualified and this book can help with that too.

Vet Nurse training across the world

While there are differences in training in each country there are many common themes. You will need to be able to:

- research and use libraries and online databases
- read critically and assess resources
- learn and retain information
- be prepared for different assessment styles
- learn to reference using an approved style.

Not all courses have a practical or work-based element and this is one of the major differences between courses. In the UK, Australia and many US states attendance in a vet practice with a structured learning path is an obligatory part of becoming a vet nurse. The way this is achieved varies: students can be employed in a practice or attend as an intern, extern or apprentice. However it is structured, there are new ways to learn and to improve your skills.

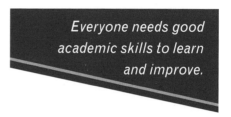

> *Everyone needs good academic skills to learn and improve.*

Regulation and the vet nurse

Where there is a requirement to attend a workplace to achieve the vet nurse qualification there is often a regulatory body for vet nurses. In the UK, this is carried out by the Royal College of Veterinary Surgeons (RCVS) who hold the register and fulfil the disciplinary duties for members of the register.

In the USA, many states have regulation for vet techs (the debate carries on about the title used, as I'm in the UK I'll use vet nurse for this book, but that includes all you vet techs too). Regulation in these states is usually carried out by the State Board of Veterinary Surgeons. In Australia, regulation is carried out by the Australian Veterinary Association and in South Africa by the South African Veterinary Association.

If you have qualified in another country and wish to move and practice in a country with a register then it is possible, and welcomed. There may be requirements to join the register and you can contact the holders of the register to find out what this requires.

You can move to many countries and travel easily with your vet nurse qualification – as long as you aren't like me and have a high maintenance dog and cat at home.

Making the most of your course

Any course that qualifies you as a vet nurse will be tough. There is a lot to learn across many diverse areas from science to customer service. There will be a variety of teaching styles and assessment styles used, not to make things harder but to provide styles of learning that suit different people.

The most commonly used assessment styles are covered in this book and I hope will help you in your personal study time. Classroom time is also important, as is making the most of your access to tutors and fellow students to improve your knowledge and skills.

To make the most of your course you need to be open to the different ways there are to learn and be assessed.

Vet nurse training makes good use of different styles of learning. Group teaching and peer learning are of great benefit, particularly for clinical skills. Many students say they do not want to learn in groups but there are many benefits and it is helpful to your progress if you can approach these sessions with an open mind.

Watching and learning from your peer group can be easier than learning from a tutor who is an experienced vet or vet nurse. Sharing revision tips and experiences of learning in practice are all important parts of your journey as a student vet nurse. You do not need to become best friends with your whole year group but being open to working with those in your group will benefit you – even if it feels difficult at first.

Here's to making success in your vet nursing course achievable and hopefully enjoyable!

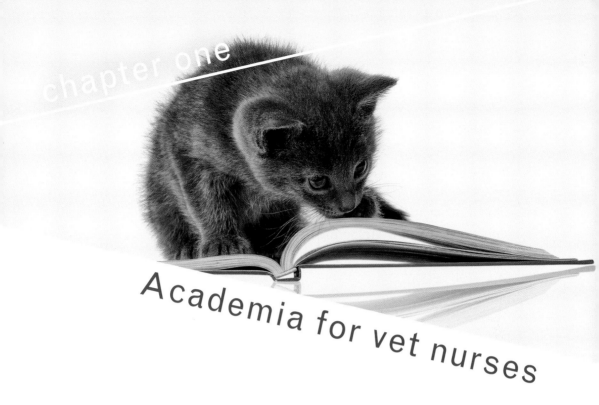

Academia for vet nurses

Why we need academic courses in vet nursing

There have been many positive changes in the veterinary nursing world in recent years. In the UK, we have protection of the title **veterinary nurse** (from the **Royal College of Veterinary Surgeons (RCVS)** through their code of conduct for vets and nurses. We can use the post nominals RVN for registered veterinary nurse and we have a professional status as we have regulation, research and training standards that befit a profession.

Vet nursing education needs to reflect these changes and to improve the skills taught to advance our profession. We now have access to several courses in the UK and abroad. In the UK, there are two routes to entering the RCVS **register** to become a **registered veterinary nurse (RVN)** and further courses for advancing having done so. We can start with a diploma or degree to qualify, diploma students can then progress to a top up degree. And we can all proceed to master's level qualifications, all within the veterinary nurse skills base.

Outside of the UK there are face-to-face and online courses in Ireland, the USA and Australia, New Zealand and South Africa, leading to

Clearly there is a need and a desire for academically skilled nursing staff for veterinary work.

a variety of vet nursing/**vet tech** qualifications. In the forthcoming book from J. Dugmore and K. Kissick *So You Want to Be a Vet Nurse?* (5M Publishing) you can find out more about the different ways to become a vet nurse in the UK and how to enter the register if you are an overseas qualified vet nurse.

The question I have heard people ask occasionally is 'why does the course have to be so academic?'. This is usually in response to either themselves or someone they know struggling to pass part of the course. It is important to bear in mind that it is a challenging course, as are all qualifications leading to a professional status. While the history of vet nurse education stems from lower-skilled care roles, such as traditional kennel maids, vet nurses are now multi-skilled medical practitioners. We can undertake medical and minor surgical procedures that require both competent practical skills and a level of theoretical understanding to be applied alongside those practical skills. Therefore, we need training courses that teach the theory and practical aspects of our roles, to improve the outcome for our patients.

This book is written to help people achieve the veterinary nursing qualification across all the assessment criteria and to take these learning and development skills into their career. Assessment styles and **learning needs** are covered in the nine chapters and learning materials are available to download for free at the webpage below and are highlighted in this book by this sign 📖.

https://www.5mbooks.com/study-skills

Providing a place to see, understand and learn all the skills to achieve and progress in a way that all can access.

We also need academic skills to support our work in practice. The profession is advancing and we have access to valuable research that can improve what we do every day. We can improve patients' care and our own self-care. To do this we need the skills to research and apply new information appropriately in our workplace. When you are asked to write a new standard operating procedure (SOP) where do you find that information? Is it reliable? And, how do you apply it to your team's **skill** levels and access to equipment? If you are in a hurry head to Chapter Nine to see more on writing a SOP.

Every time we use evidenced research to support our actions we are starting to create a better workplace, for us and for our patients. If you carry out small projects regularly you will not lose your skills for researching and producing work.

For those studying to enter the register or for post-registration qualifications it is worth writing your own guide as to how best you study. The length of your course is long enough to find this out and while our study habits change over time it is good to have a personalized guide detailing what you have found beneficial previously. This book will introduce you to activities that can help expand your learning skills repertoire.

Exam nerves

I cannot go any further with this book without addressing a problem that most of us have dealt with at some point: exam nerves.

An exam assesses your work in a 'performance', by that I mean at a set time and place. While assignments and work-based learning have a deadline, you are free to do the work at a time and place to suit you as long as the deadline is met. Exams ask you to produce the best of your knowledge in a limited time to a set criteria. You are required not just to remember facts but to apply your knowledge to discuss cases, disease processes and more.

As with any performance most people have nerves. In fact, I will go so far as to say everyone has nerves. However, some people either do not admit to them or they have such good coping strategies they can use their nervous energy as a positive force. This is something I think we can all achieve, but most of us need a little help getting there.

Every day as a vet nurse we are faced with 'performing'. We see patients in many different situations and are expected to use our knowledge to make

At work, it's like we sit mini exams all day and we don't get nervous.

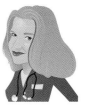

timely decisions in their best interests. Clients ask us about disease processes, treatment options or even just how flea treatments work.

This is possibly because we are in our comfort zone at work and we are confident in what we are saying. Possibly because we perceive that a client or colleague is not trying to find out what we do not know so we are confident in talking about what we do know. Either way we have the skill within us to recall information and present it in a suitable fashion – we just need to be able to do that in an exam.

What do exam nerves do to our body and brain?

We usually see nerves or being nervous as a bad thing, yet our nervous system is always trying to help us. As you will need to study anatomy and physiology let us look at a little of it now.

The autonomic nervous system controls the spinal nerves that are connected to motor function (Aspinall, 2006). These are divided into two types, the sympathetic and the parasympathetic. These names help you remember what they do. The sympathetic nervous system helps you in times of stress. It prepares your body for our two means of basic survival – we either face up to whatever the threat is or we run away; often called 'fight or flight'. This means our heart rate increases to push oxygen to our muscles so we are prepared for whichever route we take – fight or flight. Our respiratory rate increases to draw in more oxygen and stored energy is released.

We usually see nerves as a negative feeling. That increase in heart rate or breathing that we have not planned for can be scary. They are there to try to help our bodies cope with stress, and you can use this to your advantage – use that energy release for your benefit.

Preparing for being nervous

As the autonomic nervous system is not under conscious control it can feel a little overwhelming to have physical changes take place that we have not consciously chosen. What can you do to prepare for this?

An exam is a stressful situation. Even when you have revised and prepared and feel confident, you can still get nervous. That means you are likely to feel some of the sympathetic nervous system actions. This is completely normal. It is not a sign you are unprepared or have not revised enough. It is just your body reacting to an unusual situation. Recognising this helps you

The first step is to acknowledge that you might get nervous.

accept the changes and see them as a normal part of sitting an exam.

Some people never feel comfortable with the physical changes that occur. This can be for many reasons and it can stop them performing well in exams. If you feel that is you then I have some strategies to help you.

How to make nerves help us

Use your anatomy revision to help you. As a veterinary nurse, you will be able to understand that your sympathetic nervous system is trying to help you. If you relax about the changes that can occur, it helps you and if you distract yourself it can also help. You are going to have a lot to do on an exam day so distracting yourself will probably be quite easy. Finding the venue, making sure you have your paperwork or identification to register and/or log in. This will all keep you busy. You may also find an information 'hook' to help you focus on what you can recall rather than worrying about the things you cannot, more on this in Chapters Four, Five and Six.

A 'hook' is that piece of information or revision that comes easily to mind. Even if you do not need that piece of information in the exam it shows you that you can access things in your memory and that hopefully your mind will not go blank when the exam starts. This 'hook' can then be used just before and at the start of an exam to stop your brain heading off into worries about how well you will do or how calm other people seem. It takes the energy your sympathetic nervous system is providing and uses it in a positive way.

Once the exam has started your energy is usually at its highest. It is worth using this time to write down your own revision notes, even before you read the questions. This is particularly helpful for calculations in written or multiple-choice question (MCQ) exams. Once you start reading the question your brain works overtime trying to put the numbers given into the calculation, which can be confusing. To avoid this, write down the calculations on your spare paper at the start of the exam. Then when a calculation question comes up you have your own readymade crib sheet.

This can also work for any mnemonics or memory aides you have. Write them down and clear your brain space at the start of the exam. You feel more confident as you have recalled information, calming any worries your mind will go blank. You can then read the questions and plan your exam success.

Once you are distracted by these positive activities you will usually find your increased heart rate and respiratory rate will return to normal, you have used your nerves well.

If you find your heart and respiratory rates have not returned to normal or you are worried they will not then there are some breathing and focus techniques that can help. These can be of most benefit just prior to going into the exam. There are usually a number of people waiting with you and their coping strategies may not help yours. Many people use their nervous energy to get overexcited and distract themselves by talking or laughing loudly. Some try to trade information or try to guess potential exam questions, which can be off putting.

If you can focus on your own welfare that can really help you. You already have a 'hook' for your memory. You can also try focusing on the physical changes nerves bring, can you reduce your heart rate and breathing?

It is out of the scope of this book to explore all the options for calming nerves. There are so many and they need to be an individual choice. There is one simple technique that is focusing on breathing in and out. It sounds simple but it is very easy to take short shallow breaths when you are nervous and you can end up feeling unwell if this carries on for a long time. People often hold their breath reading the exam paper and we know how quickly oxygenation saturation drops when there is no breathing. This quick guide adapted from the NHS (2018) suggests the following.

- Let your breath flow as deep down into your belly as is comfortable, without forcing it.
- Try breathing in through your nose and out through your mouth.
- Breathe in gently and regularly. Some people find it helpful to count steadily from one to five. You may not be able to reach five at first.
- Then, without pausing or holding your breath, let it flow out gently, counting from one to five again, if you find this helpful.

- Keep doing this for three to five minutes.
- You may find three counts to breath in and five to breathe out is more calming than equal breathes in and out.

Three to five minutes might sound like a long time but if it gets you working at your optimum level for the whole exam it is worth it. For many people four to five breaths in and out in this manner have a positive effect and they start to relax.

If it goes wrong in the exam?

I am sure some people will read the above techniques and still feel they will not work for them. Or they have sat in exams in the past and have not been able to complete it to the level they wished.

If you get in such a situation, use your time well. Writing down a lot of things that you are not sure of or are questioning the correctness of does nothing for your confidence. This then makes you doubt everything you write, when in fact you may well be answering the questions and doing well, and may lead you to stop writing as you become so worried about what you write.

If you find yourself in this spiral, then realising you are is the first step to preventing it happening. Take time to try one of the steps above. Breathe, write down one thing that is on your mind about the question you are answering. Start with the simplest fact and more will come. No one sees your thought process so you can make it as simplistic as you like. Getting to know how your brain works is important in succeeding at learning – and knowing how your brain behaves in an exam is very important.

For example, a multiple-choice question may ask, 'In the dog, which bone articulates with the scapula distally?' You may not know the answer straight away and may need to work through your recall of the skeletal system in your own way. You can memorize the system from nose to tail, or the axial, appendicular or splanchnic systems, or working dorsal to palmar. Any way you retain or recall information is fine!

Succeeding with different needs

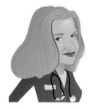

We all have different needs in our learning journey!

Identified or unidentified learning needs are no barrier to studying at a high academic level. Having a learning need can mean a physical, emotional or other issue that alters your ability to learn. Many students feel that having gotten onto the course, which was the hard part, they should not need to seek further help once they are there. While it is true that you should commend yourself for getting on a course with such high demand as vet nursing, I would encourage you to accept every bit of help offered. Seeking or making use of help offered is not a sign that you should not be on the course, instead it shows you are an emotionally mature learner who wishes to succeed. All educational establishments provide learning support and they have great information that might just help you, you just need to ask.

Emotional well-being

Learning needs can come in many forms. Some people struggle with language, some numeracy and others with the emotional and physical impact studying has. It is important to remember that many things impact on your ability to study.

As with many books on study skills, I do need to mention the things we all know but often do not prioritize – eating and sleeping well, and keeping our emotional well-being as stable as possible (Figure 1.1). These three things will help you learn as you will be in the best physical and mental state. If you are worried about your mental health, for any reason, then do please seek help. Taking on new challenges in life is stressful and vet nursing courses are no different.

Your emotional well-being is as important as eating and sleeping. Problems such as depression or low self-esteem can make learning more difficult. It

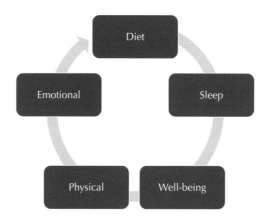

Figure 1.1 Emotional well-being cycle

is important to not be too hard on yourself and seek help if you feel you need it. Although it can be hard to acknowledge a link between the poor mental health and a lack of success with learning, especially if you have coped before.

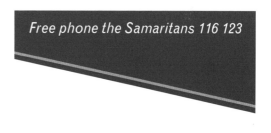

Free phone the Samaritans 116 123

If you need to talk to someone there are places to help. If you are feeling overwhelmed and need to talk to someone urgently then please call the Samaritans for free on 116 123. In the USA and Australia there are also free mental health helplines.

This is not meant to alarm you. Studying will not be so awful that you will need to seek help, but should you need to, have a number easily accessible. When you feel unwell and need help quickly then even finding a phone number to help you can feel like the biggest job in the world.

Those at college or university will find that most have access to very speedy student support. It will be on their website and sometimes on staff's email signatures. There are usually signs around campus also. However, if your course

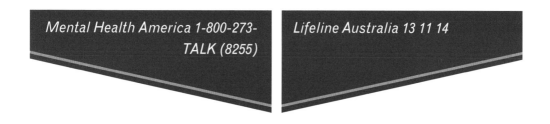

Mental Health America 1-800-273-TALK (8255)

Lifeline Australia 13 11 14

is by distance learning then you may not be on campus to see them – so use the number above if it is an urgent situation.

Vetlife 0303 040 2551

We have our own industry support line in the UK – Vetlife.org.uk 0303 040 2551. Like the Samaritans this is a 24 hour, 365 days a year service. Vetlife is specifically for vets and vet nurses and so they understand the strain of working and studying and the emotional pressure we can be under.

I hope you do not ever feel the need to call a helpline, but as mental health issues can as readily affect us as a physical ailment I would rather give you the information here and know you can access support than write a whole chapter on mental health – giving it a stigma it does not need and marking it out as separate to other issues in life, when we know it does not work like that.

Physical well-being

We know that being in the veterinary industry is physically demanding. This does not mean we should be heroes and ignore pain or use our pharmacology knowledge to treat our pain. Our health is precious, as we care for our patients' well-being then we should care for our own. This includes during our studying time.

I struggle with joint and back pain, limiting where I can work from. Many library chairs are really uncomfortable and not suitable for me. Therefore, I must plan this into my work schedule. When I am researching, I must check where I can access resources. If they are not available online, I need to check where I need to go to access them. How long the journey might be, whether I can park, and I need to consider how good the chairs are.

It sounds like a little thing but it can make all the difference between being able to concentrate and learn or finding I am distracted by pain. I can recommend the British Library chairs for support and comfort. It is important to note that this is something people will not see I am planning into my work.

Identifying and addressing your learning needs does not mean other people can see your needs.

We all learn differently

Throughout this book information and ideas will be presented to help every learner. We all have different **learning styles** and abilities. If you find some information harder to take in than others, then it is good to remember it's exactly the same for everyone else. The most successful learners are those who know what works for them and use this recognition to their advantage. They may not necessarily avoid learning in ways that they find difficult but they acknowledge the added time and work that will be needed.

The variety of assessment styles on vet nursing courses is of great benefit to all students. Having a variety of assessment styles means there will be times you are assessed in a style you prefer and do better at. As there are common areas in preparing for assessments you can play to your strengths and make every assessment style work for you. You are assessed using a mix of at least six commonly used methods:

- short-answer written exams
- long-answer written exams
- multiple-choice question exams
- seen/open book exams
- practical exams or OSCEs (objective structured clinical exams)
- work-based practical assessment (NPL or CSL)
- assignments and dissertations
- oral exams or vivas.

Some styles of assessment you are likely to have done before and some may be new. For some modules you may face written exams; other modules may be assessed through assignment or practical assessment. You do not want your grades or progress limited by the assessment style.

If you have already been identified as having a learning need it's highly likely you have an excellent idea of what works for your learning. This makes you an efficient and usually a successful student, even if some aspects of learning take you more time or effort.

Spending some time working out what learning methods work for you is not time wasted or even an attempt at procrastination. Reading this book can help make you a better learner and more likely to be successful, so do try some of the options for learning presented in the following chapters.

Many people make it through to further and higher education without receiving the full support they could have. While their own personal coping strategies may have got them onto the course of their dreams, those strategies may not be enough to succeed in the future. If you are worried about a learning need then do please speak to your college or GP and find help that you can use.

Learning styles

As part of an induction into many courses you will take a learning styles assessment. This is to help you identify your learning style. There are many tests available online and you can do them yourself if you wish.

The most commonly used tests try to put you into categories.

VAK

- V (visual) – learns best from pictures, video, infographics.
- A (auditory) – learns best from listening to information.
- K (kinaesthetic) – learns best by taking part in a **task**.

Most people are a mix of VAK, so you may find a combination of ways of learning work best for you.

Honey and Mumford

- Activist – learns by taking part in activities.
- Pragmatist – learns by placing ideas and plans into the real world.
- Theorist – learns by understanding the theory behind actions.
- Reflector – learns by taking time to review new information and consider it before putting it into practice.

These are a very basic outline of the two most popular learning styles. They are provided to give you a starting point should you wish to find out more. It is important to use the results of any assessment as a guide and check if there have been any changes to your learning style. As you mature as a learner your preferred learning styles may change. You should keep an open mind and explore as many different learning styles and opportunities as you need to.

It is also important not to see the results as labelling your personality, or saying that you will not learn in any other way. While trying to fit into a learning style 'box' can seem convenient and it is certainly a quick way to identify your needs it can be limiting.

CREAM – finding your style

There is an alternative way to find what works best for you. Cottrell (2013) advocates the CREAM strategy (Table 1.1).

I am sure you can find many other ways to keep your learning varied and interesting. We will go further into different aspects of each assessment style in the following chapters. For instance, creative memory techniques are covered in Chapters Four and Seven.

Table 1.1 CREAM strategy

C – creative	Apply creativity to your learning and problem solving.
	You could use mnemonics as memory hooks.
R – reflective	Use your own experience as a learning tool.
	You could apply experiences logged in your NPL/CSL across your theory learning.
E – effective	Be organized.
	You could learn how to search online databases efficiently.
A – active	Be engaged physically and mentally.
	You could use each study session to its fullest, be present in each session.
M – motivated	Keep clear goals for days or weeks, or for modules and deadlines.
	You could permit yourself small rewards for each goal.

Source: Cottrell (2013).

Reflection and its role in learning

What is reflection?

Reflection is a process of reviewing events and experiences and using the information to improve your performance in the future.

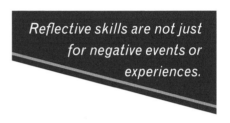

Reflective skills are not just for negative events or experiences.

Reflection bridges the gap between theory and practical learning as it involves consciously thinking and then actively making decisions (Jasper, 2003).

You should use your reflective skills for events and experiences where you would like to achieve deeper learning and to apply your theory knowledge to your clinical skills.

We need to learn to become reflective practitioners. It is a skill just like learning to use Harvard references correctly or search efficiently using an online library database. We reflect in daily life and already have basic skills to build on.

Every day we have instances where we later think 'I wish I had . . .'. This is the start of the reflective process. You have identified an experience, found something you would like to change and have an idea what that change would be.

When we do this in everyday life it is an unconscious act. How often have we thought 'I wish I had said . . .', in response to a comment or situation? It is unlikely that we will be in that situation again so while we reflect we then put it to one side and move on.

When we use reflection for improving clinical skills we know we will carry out these tasks again, perhaps repeatedly. So, we can move our reflection forward by implementing our 'I wish I had . . .' moment the next time we do the task.

How do I start reflecting?

To get the full benefit of reflection you need to be able to identify experiences and then apply them to a **reflective cycle**. There are also some short guides in Chapters Eight and Nine, which you are welcome to head straight to. However, before reading in depth about the subject let us start with the basics.

There are some commonly used terms in veterinary nurse reflection that can be used in more than one way.

Task

- Used to describe the individual aspects of work-based learning that are logged via the case based progress log (**NPL** or **CSL**).
- Also used to describe the practical examinations student nurses take. Grouping NPL/CSL tasks together in exams to reflect veterinary nursing skills.
- A piece of work that has to be undertaken (Oxford English Dictionary, 2017).

Skill

- Used to describe our practical and clinical abilities.
- Also used to describe individual or groups of tasks for the NPL/CSL.
- The ability to do something well (Oxford English Dictionary, 2017).

Experience

'Experience' is both a noun: 'an event or occurrence which leaves an impression on someone' (Oxford English Dictionary, 2017). For example, when discussing the work day with colleagues you might say, 'Cat ward was [a] great [experience] today.'

And also a verb:

- undergo an event or occurrence (Oxford English Dictionary, 2017)
- feel emotions or sensation (Oxford English Dictionary, 2017).

For example, using experience as a verb: Discussing a different day but the same ward you might say 'If cat ward is always like this I won't to do that [or *experience* that] again.'

As you can see it can be very confusing! In our veterinary nurse training, we also use the term 'experience' to name the events we log on the electronic record of cases – the NPL or CSL. This can help you focus your reflection by considering the whole skill required and where the individual task fits in.

Once you start to think through experiences, skills and tasks in this way you can start to select which to focus on. You can start to differentiate between the two experiences above.

- Was it the cat ward that was stressful or was it other factors that may appear elsewhere?
- If they appeared elsewhere what would the differences be and how could you deal with them to improve how you feel?

This is particularly helpful as a student. Where you are faced with new information and new situations on a regular basis it can feel overwhelming. You can feel like you need to reflect on everything you do, but you do not. You need to select which events to reflect on and we will now look at ways to learn how to do this.

How to use reflection in learning

In the beginning, it may help to balance reflection with reviewing two experiences at the same time. One which you felt went well and one which you felt could have been improved. Part of the reflective process could be to compare the two situations and note the similarities and differences. It is also important to consider the influences surrounding each situation.

As noted by Teekman (2000) we understand that the environment we work in and the industry we work in can affect what we do and how we reflect on it. To use reflection to learn we need to acknowledge all the factors that could affect us. We need to have as much information as possible to help us. When experiences are in a busy environment with a lot of people around, how do you start to make sense of it all?

A simple way to get started is to answer some simple questions about the situation you wish to reflect on. These questions are based on the 'six honest serving-men' that the poet Rudyard Kipling wrote about:

I KEEP six honest serving-men
(They taught me all I knew);
Their names are What and Why and When
And How and Where and Who.

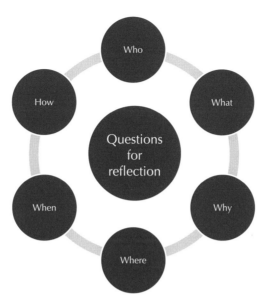

Figure 1.2 Questions for reflection

Kipling wrote this to promote using six simple questions to promote clearer thinking. It was written as part of a children's story about a baby elephant who asked too many questions – according to the adults. However, his persistence won through and there is a power shift in the story and the baby elephant and his questions are shown to be more powerful than the adults. A good reminder to never stop asking questions. The questions have been used in many ways since then and fit well with starting the process of reflection (Figure 1.2).

While reflective cycles will help you find what you need to do to move on successfully from an event, you need to learn how to select the best events to focus on to start your reflective journey.

Using these six questions will help start that process. If we go back to our original cat ward situation where the student did not want to be there again we can start to make some sense of the situation with a simple table of these questions.

The reflective table (Table 1.2) shows three columns but you could add more.

Column 1 is always going to be our starting point – the six questions.

Column 2 needs to be an accurate description of what happened. After that you can make the table into what you need. As your reflection progresses so will your table. You may find reflecting quicker and easier if you can separate the description from the reflection.

Table 1.2 Reflective table

Question	Experience information	Reflection
Who	Myself (SVN) and RVN	Usual team and have worked together before
What	Morning patient check, medicate and clean kennels	Specific issue with how I handle aggressive cats • two in ward • one with urinary catheter and IVFT
Why	Why do we do this? • clean beds if needed • clean litter trays • record over night toileting • review night shift notes • assess cats demeanour • get out of cage for assessment and administration of meds • examine IVFT, drains, catheters if needed • record findings and report to RVN and vet	I always rush cleaning to get on to more 'interesting' jobs. I hadn't thought about the process of why we clean and how important record keeping is and assessing the cats with how they respond to us. I don't think I handle the aggressive cats well as I'm rushing and they may need more time. This event has made me feel less confident.
Where	Cat ward for in-patients	18–24 patients that have been in for at least 24 hours in this ward. Stray and owned cats. All requiring medication. No boarders or healthy strays.
When	8.30 am start time	Usually takes 1–1.5 h depending on cases and staffing
How	Aggressive cat swiped me and caused me an injury. I was upset and felt I couldn't handle aggressive cats and find cat ward difficult because of this.	Looking at this list of what we hope to achieve with each cat in a short time frame I rush what we do. I didn't take time to assess the demeanour of the aggressive cat with urinary catheter and just went straight to check his urinary catheter as the bag was tangled. I should have been slower and looked at the whole patient before checking the catheter. It also is worth asking for help with cats with multiple issues as we needed to check the IVFT and the urinary catheter as well as check the bladder and carry out TPR. All of which was delayed and more difficult once he had swiped me. Reading this I realize it was not "cat ward" that was the problem but my handling of cats, in particular aggressive cats that I am a bit scared of.

Column 3 should always be filled in after column 2 – although reflection may add to your recollection and fill column 2 in more completely.

Columns 2 and 3 could also separate the event from the emotions – column 2 is what happened and column 3 is how you felt about it.

You could also add a fourth column for your plans:

- in future assess patient before opening kennel
- plan what you need to do to the patient and how you will do it before
- what situations would you ask for help in the future?

A fifth column could show where you will get further information to improve your skills:

- ask for help and advice from colleagues
- find icatcare YouTube channel for cat handling
- gain more confidence in handling with less aggressive cats.

Columns 4 and 5 could also be addressed after a discussion with your line manager or another nurse to give you a chance to reflect verbally as well as through writing.

Initially this will seem like a lot of work, but as you use tables like these they will help you begin to choose the experiences you focus on as you will begin to think of these questions while you work. These skills will help you choose which areas to reflect on.

To keep reflection positive, comparing and contrasting experiences can be beneficial. You can still use the six questions and table format, but put a positive experience and one you feel negative about side by side. It may help you if you can understand why you feel more positive about some experiences over others. Did the environment help? Was the staffing level adequate to allow for learning new skills? Was this an appropriate patient to work with when gaining confidence? All these factors impact our experiences and need to be acknowledged in our learning.

Noting external and internal factors that affect our learning is important. You may be ready to handle the unfriendly cat but if there is not a colleague there as back up or this is not the right patient then it may not be a good learning environment. This does not mean you are not capable of the task, but that this is not the right time to try your new skills and build confidence. Chapter Eight will help with the work-based learning part of vet nurse training.

Keeping reflection positive

I believe we cannot talk about reflection without mentioning mental health. It can be too easy to use reflection as a route to examining negative events in too much depth and then getting into a rut where reflection allows you to dwell on situations

> 'Self-questioning is not to be confused with self-doubt.'
> – B. Teekman

and not progress to the stages where it helps you. Reflection is a positive tool.

Teekman (2000: 1126) noted 'reflection in nurses is noted as including and centring on self-questioning – Self-questioning is not to be confused with self-doubt.'

In reviewing reflective questions asked by nurses Teekman (2000) found reflective questions were about:

- patient
- self (the nurse)
- system/environment.

These are relevant question areas to explore and can form the basis of your reflection.

It is human nature to reflect and dwell on negative events and emotions. In learning, people also think they learn the most by focusing on the areas they feel they have completed poorly. While it is true we use reflection to improve our skills and therefore we do need to review areas where we have not achieved as well as we would have liked, it is also true that even while a student it is often only a minority of events that do not go as well as we would have hoped. It is therefore important to keep in mind that while you focus on an event that was not as good as you had hoped, there were a number of other events that were positive and from which you can also learn.

Breaking down experiences with the help of the six questions, questions about your work, the patient and the environment, will all help you see there

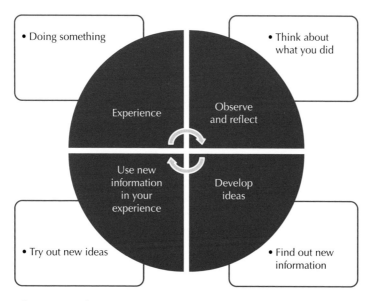

Figure 1.3 Kolb's (1984) learning cycle in Solent (2017)

are many factors in each experience and you are just one of them. If things have not gone as planned, then do not assume it has everything to do with your skills or conduct.

There is not enough space to describe the use of reflective cycles fully in this chapter – they are covered more in Chapters Three, Seven, Eight and Nine.

Once you have established the experience you wish to work on then a reflective cycle helps you 'frame' it. This means you are able to identify patterns or features in the experience that you can improve (Teekman, 2000).

While there are many reflective cycles and you can choose which one you prefer they will all follow a similar layout to **Kolb**'s cycle (Figure 1.3). As you improve with reflection you may well move onto more complex cycles that include specific areas for emotional feedback and planning for new experiences, however, as a starting point you are unlikely to feel overwhelmed by using Kolb. It leads on from the six questions and allows you to see the final step, which is taking the new information or idea you have and putting it into practice.

If we go back to the situation where the student did not want to return to cat ward, but had worked out that it was aggressive cats they were afraid of:

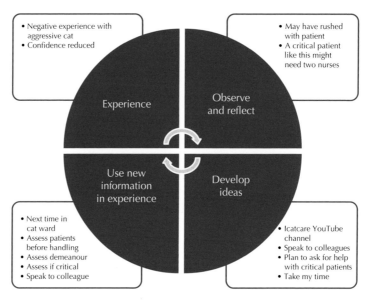

- Negative experience with aggressive cat
- Confidence reduced

- May have rushed with patient
- A critical patient like this might need two nurses

Experience

Observe and reflect

Use new information in experience

Develop ideas

- Next time in cat ward
- Assess patients before handling
- Assess demeanour
- Assess if critical
- Speak to colleague

- Icatcare YouTube channel
- Speak to colleagues
- Plan to ask for help with critical patients
- Take my time

Figure 1.4 An example of a completed Kolb's learning cycle

The reflective process is an ongoing one. Once this student has gone back into the cat ward they will then be able to reflect on their plan to improve their cat handling skills and see what works best for them in their environment.

Remember that reflection is personal to you so whatever template or table or cycle you use, make it one you find easy to work with.

Let's get started

Before you head off to the chapter you are looking for there are some things here that will help, no matter what the assessment type.

Planning and diary management

Some information will remain the same whenever or wherever you are learning. It is always worth remembering the basics about learning.

The most successful students are the ones who know their deadlines, know what is asked of them and commit to achieving that. Some may read quicker than you or do calculations faster but these skills alone are not enough.

> Success comes less from Hermione's (Harry Potter) 'books and cleverness'. And more from planning and hard work and sacrifice.

Time management and planning are key to being a successful student. Time spent planning will be saved in the future when you are working efficiently and know the deadlines and criteria for each assessment, providing the best opportunity for a successful submission.

Create a diary, either paper, on your phone or with a study diary app – there are many available for free. To create an effective planner, you need as much information as possible about what you are studying: term dates, exam dates, holidays when the library might be closed are a starting point. Then what do the exams entail – what format are they and what areas of the syllabus do they cover? When are assignments due in and are they for 3000 words or 5000 words? What about work-based learning, when does that get completed?

It is worth remembering that any vet nursing course needs a steady approach to the workload. You are more likely to thrive and succeed if you plan to achieve something every day than try to cram everything into a few long days per week. You are assessed in several ways over at least 1 year for post qualification courses and at least 2 years for **SVN** courses in the UK. You will get all the information you need to succeed in the form of a scheme of work or a term planner. But this only works for you if you read it and act on it. It is advisable to print it off and put it on your wall or screen shot it on your phone, have it somewhere you can refer to regularly – it will help. It is the basis for your diary or plan. It will show you what subjects are covered and help plan your study.

It sounds boring but it is worth it! Those people who claim to get high marks writing 3000 words in a couple of all night sessions for every deadline really are not the people to copy, or even to believe. It cannot be sustained over the length of the course.

It is a choice to treat your studying like a job; to prioritize it over other activities. Your natural abilities to read quickly or retain information easily are only useful if you actually open books and journals and read them. For that to happen you need to

> As Dumbledore says, 'It is our choices, Harry, that show what we truly are, far more than our abilities.'
> – J.K. Rowling, Harry Potter and the Chamber of Secrets

plan to search databases or head to the library. You need to know your subject areas and what assessments are coming up.

To help you plan you should consider the different ways we learn. If you have 3 hours of time to study it is unlikely you can study new subject matter in depth for the full 3 hours. To make the best use of chunks of time create a 'to do' list and vary what you are doing if you can. Consider reviewing some lecture notes or revision notes as this will be familiar material. To learn new information, you may need to read and make notes on what you have read. This is more in-depth learning and will take more time and energy. It may also create its own 'to do' list as you need to look up new words or terminology, or find more information to read. In the example in Figure 1.5 I have varied my tasks between reviewing the familiar, researching and writing about new information and planning for new lectures.

How much should you study for each module? It is natural to spend more time on areas we enjoy or find easier, and less on those we do not enjoy – but try to spend time where it is needed. There is a rough guide to how many hours you should spend on a module. If a module is worth 60 credits (Northedge, 2005) this translates to 600 hours of work. This is then spread over the time you have for the module, which may be one or two semesters.

These hours don't include breaks, chats in the library or making tea.

Mon 9 Jan 2017	
09:00 10:00	Review lung function notes
10:00 10:30	Essay – question/word count/dea…
10:30 11:00	Essay – lecture notes check
11:00 11:15	Break
11:15 12:15	Essay – library database search
12:15 12:45	Essay – online database search
12:45 13:30	Swim and lunch

 Figure 1.5 Example of a daily study planner

Generally, full-time higher education (degree) students study the equivalent of 120 credits per year, which works out at around 40 hours per week.

Making notes in lectures and from books

Note taking has come full cycle. Where pen and paper were shunned in favour of pre-printed notes we now see students taking notes via tablets, using writing-to-text software with digital pens. Whichever method you choose making notes is an active learning task and one which is very important.

However you chose to do it, making notes is a skill and one you can tailor for your exact needs, with just a few simple rules.

* Use your own words to avoid plagiarism and to develop an understanding.
* Develop your own abbreviations and acronyms.
* Use Latin abbreviations, for example, TID.
* Use lists, mind maps and spidergrams.
* Use headings and mark out subject areas.
* Annotate pre-printed notes and handouts.
* Include the date, lecture title, module and tutor.
* Include the learning outcomes covered.

You can experiment as much as you need to. You may find a linear approach of lists of information and bullet points helps you (I do!), or a more visual approach with mind maps and diagrams is better. Just remember to make sure all the notes you produce are legible and that they contain enough information when filed so you can find them again easily.

Each set of notes needs to include the module title and tutor's name. Ideally including contact details so you have easy access if you need to ask questions. The date and name of the session should also be included. Most modules will move chronologically and lectures will follow on from one another. It is also important to note what a lesson or study period is covering from your learning outcomes. A learning outcome is stated as part of a course and is usually stated in module handbooks and at the start of lessons. It can be easy to skip over these and think you will know when it has been covered and what parts of the course relate to it, but that is not always the case. Assessments are written to ensure you demonstrate understanding of the learning outcomes so make sure you know what the learning outcomes are, what parts of the course they relate to and that you understand them. You may find the exam checklist in Chapter Five helpful and also the definitions of exam wording in the same chapter – they are also in the glossary.

These rules should be followed regardless of how you record notes and how you store them, paper files can be as easy to mix up as electronic files.

To make notes from lectures easier to understand you can use a system known as **Cornell notes**. This is where you have a template with sections to complete with the information and ideas generated by a lecture. This includes

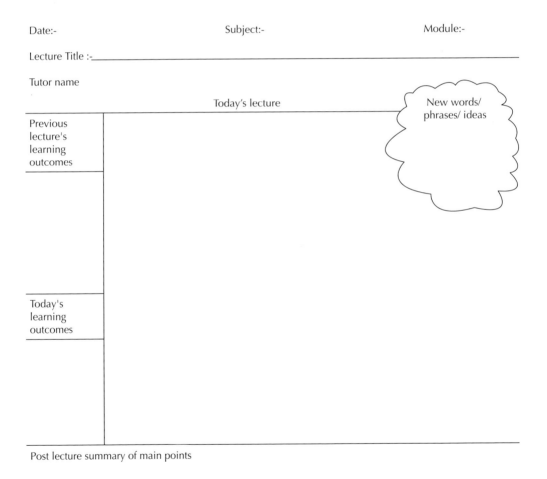

Figure 1.6 Lecture notes (adapted from Cornell)

areas that are new to you and for which you will need to find out more and it also includes writing a short summary of the lecture. This will make you write up in your own words the information you have been given, which is an important part of the learning process. An example of an amended Cornell system is shown in Figure 1.6

You can create a template for lecture note-taking based on this system that suits you. You should have several sections to add to your notes and this can be done with different boxes as in Figure 1.6 or using different coloured pens or highlighters to show where the information is in each of the sections:

- summary of the lecture
- learning outcomes covered
- ideas from previous lectures
- ideas that are new
- areas for further research.

Starting with the summary of the lecture you can use the example of the One Minute Paper (Figure 1.7) (Center for the Enhancement of Learning & Teaching, n.d.). This is a technique usually used by lecturers to help students sum up what they have learned in a lecture but there is no reason not to use it for your own summary of the lecture.

One Minute Paper
What are the most significant things you have learned during this session?
What remains uppermost in your mind?
Is there anything you did not understand?

 Figure 1.7 One Minute Paper

You should also make notes when reading text books and academic papers. You can follow a similar pattern to those notes you make from lectures. However, as you control the speed and depth with which you make these notes you can make different levels of notes depending on their use.

Overview

- a summary of a topic or subject area
- this may raise more questions that you need to answer
- it helps put big ideas into manageable chunks
- it helps you write down what you mean in your own words.

Basic introductory info

- reminders of main issues to kick start revision
- learning outcomes covered
- helps you stop going off topic.

Key points – facts, figures

- useful in planning assignments.

In depth

- can be used as the start of an assignment
- leads to a deeper understanding of the subject area
- explores differing points of view. (Northedge, 2005)

While making notes it is worth considering keeping several other supporting documents running.

Bibliography

- a list of the material you have read during your study
- useful when writing assignments and dissertations.

Reference list

- a list of all the sources of information cited in an assignment or dissertation
- must be included to provide tutors with access to the information you have found and used and to avoid plagiarism
- Where did you find the information – was it in the library, on a database, from lecture notes? How did you access it? Online, visit library, reference only, take book home, have to order, open access.

You can have each of these as separate documents on your computer or in a notebook. They will mean you can always find where you got your information and how to access it again. It also makes your reference list less of a chore for an assignment as you have the information in one place and just need to ensure it is properly formatted for your course provider's preferred style.

Organising your notes is essential, there is little point in creating useful notes if you cannot later find them. It is usually easiest to organize your notes according to the way your course is structured. Courses may focus information in weekly formats across a module, or focus on an organ or a disease as a topic. Make sure you label your notes, whether hand written or electronic, with dates and titles of lectures, topics and modules. It will mean you can find them easily when the deadlines for exams and assignments arrive.

Saving your work

You will find most colleges will not accept a technical issue as a reason for late or non-submissions of work. The need to regularly and safely keep your work is therefore *very* important. Hard drives fail, memory sticks get lost and clouds can be inaccessible.

As a minimum, I would save your work in three different places.

There are a number of options so pick what suits you best:

- computer hard drive
- external hard drive
- memory stick
- cloud-based systems
- computer back up programme
- paper copies.

I have saved this book in four places – an external hard drive, a memory stick and two cloud-based storage systems. I decided to avoid using my laptop hard drive, as if there are any laptop issues my work is safe elsewhere. Luckily, I have only had to re-set the operating system on my laptop but I have colleagues who have had their laptop stolen and they had not saved their work elsewhere; not just the loss of a laptop but all their work too.

I also keep my external hard drive and memory sticks in separate places, I am not paranoid, honestly, but if we are burgled they can have the laptop, but I do not want them to get my work as well.

The advantages of such an approach are obvious. The only real disadvantage is that it takes a little bit of time to back up each document at the end of a session and if you have a lot to store you may need to pay for a large hard drive or extra cloud storage capacity. You also need to update all the saved locations if you have been working from cloud-based versions. I sometimes work this way when in the library. I take my iPad® to save carrying my laptop and then can only save work to the cloud, so I update the hard drive and memory stick once I am back home.

You are then very unlikely to lose all of your work easily – something to bear in mind – it is better to prevent the problem than try to cure it once it has happened.

The difference between exams and essays

It is important to realize the difference between what examiners are looking for in answers to exam questions and essay questions. In essays or assignments, it is expected that you will have taken time to explore all the possible view points and have reviewed and read a number of related texts. You are expected to write substantially, usually a few thousand words, and to reference your resources. The work is set in advance and you have several weeks or more to prepare your work. You are producing a detailed view on the information available.

In exams, you may need to write a few hundred words to cover the question asked and keep within the time limit. You are not expected to reference your work or quote exact figures. You will be assessed on the information and the ideas you have presented. You are not penalized for not writing down everything you have learnt about the subject, you have neither the time or space for this in an exam. The examiner wants to see you provide information and also ideas and opinions that show you understand the question set. In Chapter Five we will look at how exam questions are set and how best to answer them.

We are sometimes so focused on showing everything we have learnt we often leave an exam thinking about what we did not write rather than what we did write. I can still recall leaving my final nursing practical disappointed I had not been asked about instrumentation as I knew that section well. I still passed my exams but wanted to parade my knowledge.

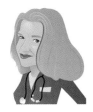

> *Don't let those feelings cloud what you actually DID in an exam and let those feelings put you off studying for further exams.*

Critical thinking

As you progress in to the higher levels of education you will find a move away from learning facts to repeat, or learning by rote, to being asked to evaluate information and make arguments for or against statements or situations.

This skill can be classed under the general term **critical thinking**. We use this skill when reading, writing, listening and when searching for new information. Cottrell (2013) uses Edward Glaser's definition to define three areas of importance.

- Persistence – consider an issue carefully and on more than one occasion.
- Evidence – evaluate the evidence put forward for the point made.
- Implications – what will follow if you uphold the viewpoint on the evidence given? Is the outcome suitable or rational? If not, should the issue be reconsidered?

This might seem a lot to consider when we are also dealing with a lot of new information. Why should we stop to decide if what we are finding out is relevant or is well supported by evidence? Surely if a paper has been published it must be good?

There is a lot of information out there for you to find and use in research and revising. Carrying out your own research is one of the main learning areas of further and higher education. How good the information you find is will depend on your research skills and your ability to evaluate the resources you find.

We use some level of critical thinking every day without really realising it. You do already have skills to build on. We are aware that newspapers report facts and opinions differently. Roughly speaking, newspapers are divided into tabloids and broadsheets. This distinction is about more than physical presentation of the newspaper, it is also a comment on the intellectual level of the writing and use of language. It is said that you need the reading ability of an 7–9-year old to read the *Sun* and that of a 14-year old to read the *Financial Times* (Media First, n.d.). The way stories are reported varies according to each newspaper's style. Tabloids are often considered to be less trustworthy than broadsheets, although many are owned by the same media companies.

You have already made a decision when you pick up a newspaper or open a news app about what you are looking for. Quick, easy to read articles or in-depth pieces with information and debate.

It is similar when finding out information while studying. Even if a study has been published you still need to examine the evidence before you.

Persistence

- Does the point of view or argument make sense?
- Does the argument follow a logical path?
- If you look at the argument from another point of view is it still logical?
- Have events since the author's point of view was formed changed the information?

Evidence

- Does the evidence provide help?
- How old is it?
- Who wrote/created it?
- Were they asked to write by anyone who could influence the evidence?

Implications

- If you decide the evidence is appropriate can you apply it to all relevant situations?
- Will the outcome in all situations be relevant and logical?

We will go into critical thinking in reading, writing and listening in future chapters. But for now, here's an example of a piece of writing to which you could apply the above questions.

Dogs suffer from tail injuries every year. In 1988 vets recorded 11% of injuries in dogs were to do with their tail (Brown, 1988). While we have traditional breeds that are 'docked' if they are working to prevent injury, it is the undocked breeds who suffer. Vets say Labradors and Staffordshire Bull Terriers often have tail injuries, yet have not been considered as breeds to dock.

Tail injuries can be hard to treat as bandages do not always stay on and the dogs continue to wag their tails. It costs the owner money and the dogs suffer.

Could the veterinary industry be preventing suffering by offering to dock tails on susceptible breeds when they are neutered? This would reduce the cost to the owner and only lengthen the surgery time by a small amount.

Mock Vet News – Jane Davidson 2017

Reference

Brown, D. (1988) *Preventing All Suffering: Is it Possible?* London: New Age Press.

How does this argument stand up to critical thinking? Although it is made up it is very similar to articles written about animal welfare.

Persistence

- How would the 89% of pet owners and dogs feel that do not have tail injuries if they were required to dock their dog's tail?
- Is 11% of dogs suffering an injury enough to justify all dogs undergoing this procedure?

Evidence

- The evidence is quite old, certainly older than the advised 5–10 years for academic works.
- Is the publisher a scientific publisher?
- Does the title of the book appear to be a veterinary title or an academic one?
- Is the use of the word suffering used factually or emotively?

Implications

- If we then noted that 12% of cats get scratched in their eyes during a cat fight should we:

    (a) keep all cats indoors on their own
    (b) remove all cats' eyes to prevent future suffering?

This may seem a rather unusual line of thought but you need to keep your critical thinking hat on when assessing new information. While on paper this may seem an easy case of an emotive argument, if you had heard someone passionately pleading the case for the poor tail-injury dogs it may be harder to spot. You have not got the opportunity to go back and check that only 11% of dogs are affected, or to see that the evidence is quite old and possibly not from a scientific source.

Becoming an SVN: the legal aspects

Even before you have started a course you might have realized there are some differences between being a student and being a student vet nurse (SVN) or vet tech. Boyd (2014) has noted that nursing students feel they are not like other students because they:

- are on placement, which is a full-time job
- have professional responsibilities of patient welfare
- are accountable for their own actions
- have a lot to learn
- are doing a physically and mentally demanding role.

While the title SVN is specific to the UK the issues of student vet nurse/tech identity are common across all courses. Some courses teach alongside vets for some of the time and then move to nursing-focused modules, some teach alongside human nurses and some courses are delivered fully online with other vet nurses/techs so you create your community in a different way.

Veterinary nursing students in the UK can feel different to other undergraduate or diploma students. Even your title as a student vet nurse sets you apart. Your role in patient care and as part of the veterinary team is acknowledged by the Royal College of Veterinary Surgeons (RCVS) and by an amendment to the Veterinary Surgeons Act 1966 (RCVS, 2002).

While SVNs in the UK are not under the jurisdiction of the disciplinary committee of the RCVS the system of regulation is taught as part of the syllabus and students need to be aware of the responsibilities they will have when qualified. During your time as an SVN you should familiarize yourself with the **Code of Conduct**.

The Code of Conduct (RCVS, 2015) was updated in 2015 and is regularly reviewed. You are identified as a student veterinary nurse if you meet the following criteria:

> Student veterinary nurses are those enrolled with the RCVS for the purpose of training at an approved centre or practice. (RCVS, 2015)

Therefore, you are only regarded as a student veterinary nurse if you have a place at an approved college and in an approved **training practice (TP)**.

The areas you need to be aware of for your time in practice and for work-based learning assessments concern delegation of duties and who is supporting and observing you. This is especially pertinent for schedule III (**SIII**) procedures.

SIII includes minor surgery, such as entering the lumen of a vein. If you are undertaking blood sampling or placing a catheter for intravenous fluids then you need to adhere to the Code of Conduct rules for direct, continuous and personal supervision:

> Direct, continuous and personal supervision means that the veterinary surgeon or veterinary nurse is present and giving the student veterinary nurse his/her undivided personal attention. (RCVS, 2015)

You are always working under the direction of a veterinary surgeon. While you are learning new skills, supervision should be direct and constant and provided by a vet or registered vet nurse. As you progress you will find the supervision required diminishes as you improve. Using the systems available to record your case by case progress you will be required to reflect on your progress. It is through this reflection that you will be able to see how you are improving in your practical skills.

In the USA, individual states license, certify or register vet techs and the state board decides its requirements, with many having similar CPD or CE (continuing education) requirements to the UK.

In Australia vet nurses are able to register in Western Australia but this is not required in other states. South African vet nurses are regulated by the South African Veterinary Association.

Starting your learning journey

Chapter One has contained a mix of information. Some as an introduction to future chapters and some you will need to access again. You may read the book through from start to finish, or dip in and out to sections and chapters as you need them. Remember there are free learning materials online too at:

> 'It matters not what someone is born, but what they grow to be.'
> – J.K. Rowling, Harry Potter and the Goblet of Fire

 http://www.5mbooks.com/study-skills

Review Chapter 1 and how to apply what you have learned with the Reflective Template.

Chapter 1 glossary

code of conduct – regulatory rules in the UK

Cornell notes – a systematic way of taking notes developed by Walter Pauk at Cornell University

critical thinking – the skill to assess information and documents that you may find and decide if they are valid resources

CSL (clinical skills log) – a digital record of cases encountered in training and reflective comments on the process

Kolb, David – published his experiential learning theory in the 1980s and developed the Kolb reflective cycle, which is still widely used today

learning needs/differences – the different emotional, physical and intellectual situations that may affect a student's ability to learn, which may be temporary, permanent, identified or unidentified, anything that means a student's learning journey differs from others

learning styles – different ways in which we may learn information

NPL (nursing progress log) – a digital record of cases encountered in training and reflective comments on the process

RCVS (Royal College of Veterinary Surgeons) – UK regulator of vets and vet nurses

reflection – the process of considering your thoughts and actions, to improve them in the future

reflective cycle – a model that can help you move through reflection to a constructive outcome, such as Kolb's

register – central record of approve practitioners, such as those held by the RCVS in the UK and by state boards in the USA

RVN (registered veterinary nurse) – a vet nurse in the register in the UK

SIII (Schedule III) – the RCVS bye-law that permits minor surgical tasks to be carried out by RVNs in the UK

skill – term used in the UK to describe the accumulation of case-based experience for student vet nurses

SVN – a student vet nurse in the UK who is registered with the RCVS and has a place at a registered training practice

task – term used in UK work-based learning to identify small parts of an overall skill

training practice – a UK vet practice that is recognized by the RCVS as a place to train vet nurses

vet tech/veterinary technician – US name for a vet nurse, regulated in some states and may be called: LVT licensed; CVT certified; RVT registered.

veterinary nurse – legal title for those who are on the RCVS register in the UK, also used in Australia and South Africa and in some states in the USA

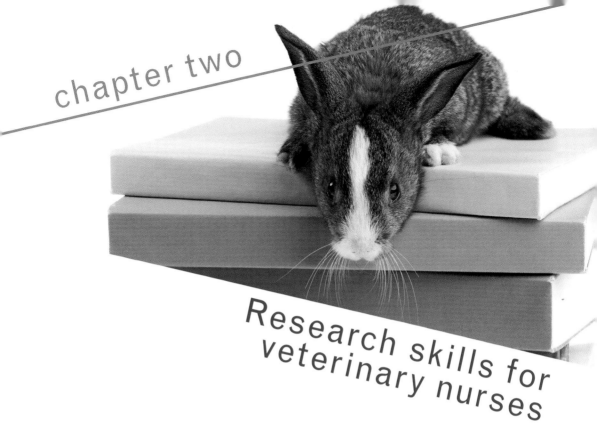

Research skills for veterinary nurses

When studying at an advanced level a significant amount of time is spent on your own, carrying out research. You may be seeking information to help you understand something that came up in lectures or to prepare for an assessment that is due. Later in your career you may need to find evidence to back up your practice's protocols, for an academic article you are writing or for some CPD you wish to provide for colleagues.

It is important you have an efficient and productive way of searching for and accessing information. While free online **search engines** enable us to access information from around the world on any number of topics instantly, they also raise issues with how to find the best information when there is so much to search through. Your research skills also need to include **critical thinking** to ensure that you locate reliable **resources** that are worth reading and citing in your work and that will add to your understanding of the subject area. How are your **digital literacy**

> 'All we have to decide is what to do with the time that is given us.'
> – *J.R.R. Tolkien*, The Fellowship of the Ring

skills: you may be able to spot 'fake news' on Facebook, but can you tell if the article you found online is good enough to use for the academic level you wish to achieve?

Whatever the source of the new information we find, we should take note of what we did to access it. When we do not know something sometimes we panic; referring back to previous research strategies will remind you how to go about researching. We all experience times when it feels like there is so much new information that we know nothing and we are undertaking an impossible task. There are times when you feel that you do not know the questions to ask to get the information that you need. Then there are the gaps where you do not know what you do not know. How do you even begin?

Strauss et al. (2010: 17) has noted different levels of knowledge.

Three levels of knowledge that we have when studying:

- Cognitive resonance – what we do know and can recall.
- Cognitive dissonance – what we know we should know but do not/ cannot recall.
- The gaps where we did not know there was something to know.

Identifying patterns in your learning will make you more able to cope with the information you do not yet know and how you will process it. Gaps in knowledge are nothing to be scared of. Acknowledging they exist and working to fill those gaps is the important step.

Some gaps in your knowledge may be created by the different depths or types of knowledge you have. It is sometimes a case of connecting the different levels of learning you already have. For example, you may know the pancreatic functions of a cat from learning by rote. However, rote learning may make applying your knowledge when understanding the disease process of diabetes in cats more difficult, as this requires application of knowledge and problem solving, which are not always a logical progression from learning by rote. You need to be able to research to find evidence that suits you and the level you are working at to connect what you already know with what you are learning.

'It is not the strength of the body, but the strength of the spirit.'
– J.R.R. Tolkien

All veterinary nursing courses are hard. Even if you have studied at the same academic level before, the depth and breadth of subject areas covered and the need to complete work-based learning at the same time make this a demanding area to study in.

As well as ensuring you have great research skills, which is what this chapter is all about, it is also worth identifying your study comfort zone. This is a logical next step from your learning style (Chapter One): finding which type of information is the best starting point for your research in any given area. Books, journals, lecture notes, videos, podcasts – which is best for you?

Finding a comfortable starting place is a good idea. By comfortable I mean either in a place or a **medium** that feels right for you. That may mean heading to the library and your 'go to' textbook as a start, or looking up key words in a veterinary dictionary. Perhaps your preferred veterinary nursing journal or veterinary newspaper have an article? Alternatively, a Google search to see what you can find, or perhaps education channels on YouTube or podcasts may help you.

As your learning journey progresses you may change what you are comfortable with, as your skills improve and the facilities available to you change. Use this chapter to improve your research skills, it will cover reading effectively, which are better – books or the internet, and how to find resources, including how to search online efficiently. It will also look at using Google to get better results, we know you will use Google, but should you?

Reading effectively

You may be tempted to skip this section. I know I would think twice about being told about something as basic as 'how to read'. But this is not about how

> *Reading effectively allows you to succeed when it feels like the information is written in a different language.*

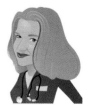

to read your favourite novelist in a better way, it is about how to approach reading academic work.

Critical reading – ensuring validity

While starting with material from your preferred medium is a great goal and one to use to find material you understand easily, you also need to look for other sources of information. As we mentioned in Chapter One you need critical reading skills. Your time is precious so you want to make sure that the work you read is the best possible available for the subject area. Just as you would do in everyday life you want to make sure you can trust the information given (see Figure 2.1). While as an introduction to a subject area videos or podcasts are helpful, at the time of writing, you are still going to find most of your academic resources are **journal** papers or books.

Before you start reading the content of work you find, it is important to find out a bit more about how it was published. This might sound like adding more to your workload, however, there is very little point in reading an article or

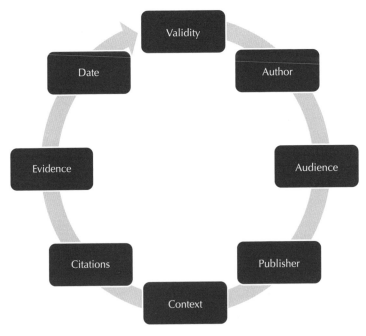

Figure 2.1 Factors affecting the validity of academic writing

chapter in depth to find it was published 15 years ago, or to discover in later reading that the author's ideas were disproved in future research. You can avoid both of these by doing some basic checks and referring back to the critical thinking section of Chapter One.

To check if the information you are reading is valid and worth your time, draw up a checklist of some or all of the following items and quickly assess each piece of information against it (see Figure 2.1).

Author – who are they?

- Are they known in their field?
- You may need to search for some more information on them.
- Do not rely on them being a familiar name to guarantee that they are the best source for the particular field you are researching.

Audience – who was it written for?

Is it for vets, students, veterinary specialists or pet owners? This will help you decide if it will have information that is relevant to your research.

Publisher/journal type

Aim for academic journals, preferably those that use **peer review**, such as *The Veterinary Nurse, the Journal of Small Animal Practice* and other similar titles. While trade papers, such as the *Vet Times,* may have the most up-to-date news and may be an easy way to start research, you should use them as a gateway to other evidence rather than hanging an entire argument on an article that has not been peer reviewed and may have been published as a 'point of view' or personal interest piece with few references to back it up.

Context

Consider whether the research was paid for by a third party? Research funding regularly comes from grant providers and commercial interests, such as drug companies and feed/supplement providers, you should be aware of this and plan to find research that cannot be accused of being biased.

Additionally, was the article or chapter written in response to an earlier piece and is it an ongoing debate? With some debates, you might need to read preceding papers to fully understand what it is being argued. This is particularly true around subjects such as the use of homeopathy, and the protection of the veterinary nurse title, where opinions are divided.

Citations

When researching online databases, you regularly see statistics on how many people have used a work to support their own academic writing. An article with a high number of **citations** would seem a good choice as it is popular.

However, you should consider such popularity. People may be citing the work as it is relevant and a positive contribution or they may be citing it as a poor example of work or data and be criticising it. It is also hard to see if it is being cited in the field you are researching. It may be cited in another field entirely – for example, you may be looking for data on the prevalence of hyperthyroidism in cats over 10 years' old, but the paper may actually be cited regularly for its information on nutrition for older cats. While this may overlap with your research area the high level of citations does not mean it is the best paper for your work.

Evidence offered

Does the evidence provided and the conclusion drawn make sense? Is the **reference** list mainly recent academic journals that would also pass your critique?

Date – how old is too old?

You will be encouraged to use references that are under 10 years' old. If you are submitting work in 2018, the papers and books should be published no later than 2008. Yet this has its limitations.

Some core textbooks can take several years to write and edit and may only be published or updated every 8 to 10 years. But they are still relevant as they are key texts in teaching. Articles are quicker to write and publish and so should really be no older than 5 to 10 years.

However, this also depends on the subject area. Some areas of veterinary nursing may have had limited new research published within the last 5 years.

This is because it is a relatively young profession and the amount of research available is limited, albeit growing.

It is not necessarily wrong to cite work older than 5 to 10 years. There may not be much newer evidence. However, if your citations are all over 5 years old you should put a brief explanation to show you understand your resources and reflect on any needs for further research if appropriate. You should also be wary of citing only very recent work. While some research areas will seem very exciting because they have a lot of new evidence you will very likely have to cite older evidence to explain how and why recent advances have occurred. It is best practice to acknowledge the age of resources, if there is a prevalence for older or newer works, and to explain why this may be.

Conclusion

Does the conclusion follow on from the evidence presented? Does it make sense? If the evidence does not support the conclusion, then it is not a suitable resource.

This is a lot of information to consider (see Figure 2.2). We can make it easier by thinking of our questions from reflection. Always keep a critical mind when viewing work, even when published in reliable journals.

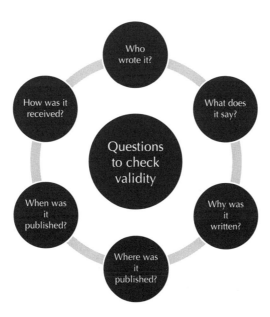

Figure 2.2 Questions to check validity

This is a lot of information to check. How can you ensure you do not miss anything? Northedge (2005: 238) has a simple mnemonic:

- P   presentation – does it look professional?
- R   relevance – is it medical, nursing, veterinary?
- O   objectivity – is there any bias?
- M   method of research
- P   **provenance** – who wrote it and why?
- T   timeliness – was it published within last 5 to 10 years?

Once you have decided the information is worth a closer look then you need to consider how best to spend your time. To assess information you will need to scan papers and chapters quickly and accurately, read on to see how to do that.

Speed reading

You may already be familiar with the differences between speed reading and reading in depth. Speed reading can be used to preview information by getting a brief view of what it contains and to work out if it's something worth spending more time on later. Reading in depth will give you a better understanding of the subject matter. Both are needed to further your research and learning.

Boyd (2014) notes two different ways of speed reading. Scanning and skimming.

Scanning

Scan read the text and focus on:

- introduction and conclusion
- first and last paragraphs of the main body of the text
- check for headings/chapter titles that may be of interest and read the first paragraph under that heading (for example, if you are looking for positive information on raw feeding if you scan the headings you may find that as an article or chapter heads to a different viewpoint it is not as helpful an article as it seemed).

Skimming

Skimming is best achieved by picking out headings and key words that you are looking for.

- Skim the whole text in a methodical manner working from introduction to conclusion.
- If not finding your key words frequently, note which words similar to your key words are present (if any). For example, if you are looking for information on acute renal failure in cats then you may find your search brings you information about chronic renal failure as well. Some articles or chapters may discuss some aspects of both together so scan reading will quickly let you identify which parts are relevant to your search.

The scanning style of speed reading is better suited to textbooks as it does not require you to read the whole text, but focus on the areas of interest. As books can cover a large subject area, it may only be part of a chapter that is relevant to your search. This does not mean it is less valid than an article that is solely dedicated to your preferred subject area, it just requires a different approach to find it.

Using speed reading to read academic text is a great starting point: use it to find out if the text is worth more of your time. The next step is to note any unfamiliar words or phrases and find out what they mean, this will also help you decide if it is worth more of your time. You can then start in depth reading.

In depth reading

In depth reading is discussed in detail by Northedge (2005). He notes that reading in depth is a skill that needs to be learned. It will also take time and energy and will use active reading skills. You need a plan.

- Find out what new words mean – keep a list and look up meanings using an appropriate dictionary. While there are numerous reliable ones online, having a veterinary dictionary to hand is very useful.

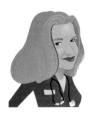

Reading academic work is not like reading an article in a celebrity magazine (not that I read those, obviously!)

- Make your own dictionary of terms, phrases and words that you need to understand. This can be using a notebook, flashcards or creating your own electronically. You can collate this alphabetically from beginning to end or you could create mini-dictionaries grouped around subject areas.
- Simplify key arguments into your own words. If you find the information hard to take in because the author's wording is complex, then try to explain it as if you were speaking to someone with no veterinary knowledge, this will reinforce your understanding of it.
- Forgive the academic style. It is not to put you off, but to make exacting arguments accurately and with little chance of misunderstanding. It can come across as a very 'dull' way to write. But it has its purpose, to present as much information and evidence as possible in a coherent manner and not to include anything that does not add to the stated viewpoint.
- Set up a suitable environment to work in. Quiet and comfortable with space to spread out your paperwork.

You can also use in depth reading to help improve your recall of information. Boyd (2014) has suggested using the 'SQ3R' process: survey, question, read, recall, review.

Survey, question, read, recall, review

This is where you survey, or scan read some information first. From this you can formulate some questions that you would like to answer from the information provided. Then you read and try to find the answers to your questions. If you do find answers then you note them down and later try to recall the answers without looking at your notes or the text. The final stage is then reviewing that what you recalled is correct and meets your needs for the assessment you are aiming for. While this is more aimed at revising for exams so you can recall information, it can be used in determining the relevance of information you are reading.

In depth reading is a slower process than many people think. You are working hard to learn and understand new information on a deeper level. You may also want to incorporate active note making in your reading. We have covered note making in Chapter One so please revisit that if you need to remind yourself of some tips.

As you do more in depth reading you will find a way that suits you best. As you do, your ability to learn new information will improve. To see how well you are working, set yourself targets and monitor whether you improve, or whether you prefer different authors or types of information presentation,

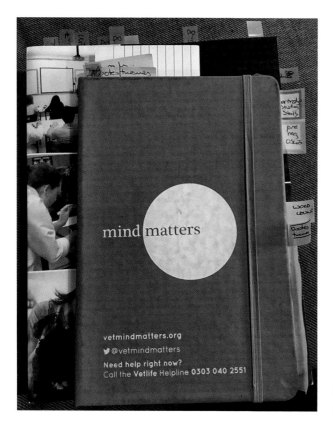

Figure 2.3 Sticky notes marking relevant reading

for example, tables, linear notes, infographics, or writing styles particular to certain journals or books. Additionally, once you start your academic writing you will need detailed reading skills to edit your own work effectively, so it is important to build these skills.

Even if you improve your skills you may still find you struggle to read certain authors or styles of writing. It is important to not get blocked or stuck on a paragraph or page. If you do not understand what is being said, then scan read to the next page to see if an overview of the topic as a whole makes that particular section make sense. If it still does not help, look at other information on the subject that is presented in a different way. This may help break through the block you are having in this area.

Active reading

Active reading is the step before going to make notes and you may find you use both ways of reading together or separately as part of a study plan. Active reading involves marking text passages with highlighters or underlining sections. It also includes making notes to reflect ideas you have or questions you need to answer.

If you do not own the text you wish to mark up you can use sticky notes, which can be removed later before returning the text. These come in a variety of sizes, colours and styles to suit whatever you need. You may wish to use the larger ones to draw visual aids or to write information in your own words. Sticky notes are also very useful in texts you do own to flag up content. Figure 2.3 shows one of my note books, with sticky notes to mark pages.

Keep your active reading challenging by asking yourself questions about your notes.

- Do you understand what the author is saying?
- Does this link to anything you already know?
- Do you have any further knowledge gaps to fill?

Working with numbers – how to use them in critical reading

Many student nurses have said to me 'I'm no good at maths' and I always point out the following.

- Working with numbers is key to what we do.
- There is a difference between numeracy and maths.
- Numeracy is what we do every day.

Maths is the thing we learn at school, which is the knowledge of different forms of working with numbers – algebra, Pythagoras and all those things we cannot quite recall. Maths is working to find out the answer for the purpose of solving a problem or proving an equation works.

Numeracy is different. Numeracy is having numerical literacy, being able to work with numbers in your daily life. From working out where has the best offers for the food you buy to calculating household bills. It also works in the workplace, it is the skill you use to work out a drug dose rate. Or the ability to read a graph or table to give the appropriate amount of food.

In assignments, you will need to be able to read tables as part of your scan reading and also to access the data in them when reading in depth. They can help you spot valid or invalid information. When reading tables Northedge (2005) has some simple tips.

- Read the information about the data – headings, axis, names.
- Scan for highest and lowest figures in each column, bar, graph.
- See if there are any patterns/anomalies.
- Write down what it shows in your own words.

This will show you if the data given is of interest to you. If you were trying to find research on preventing hypothermia in cats during surgery by using blankets you would be interested in a table showing pre- and post-operative temperature readings.

You would want to know what they had used to cover the cat to get the different readings. Then scanning for highest and lowest temperatures would quickly let you see if there were any clear improvements with any of the types of blankets.

Patterns then start to show. Did young cats respond best, was the length of surgery a factor? Writing down these brief points in your own way will help as you may list them then from best performing to worst performing and allow you to start reading the paper with this information in mind. There is more information on reading charts and tables in Chapter Five.

Producing your own research – graphs and charts

You may have to produce evidence of your own research during your studies. You will need to display the results of primary research you have carried out, for example, responses to a questionnaire or data from experiments carried out.

A graph or bar chart is usually better than a table as it is an easily readable visual display of data. Graphs also allow readers to predict future trends based on your findings (Northedge, 2015). If the data set is large or complex, providing the raw data used to create a graph or chart in an appendix table or as a downloadable resource is a good way to fully support your conclusions while avoiding clogging up the presentation.

There is a huge variety of software available to let you do this and it should not become an exhaustive part of writing up your evidence. Microsoft products such as Word and Excel allow data to be presented in graphs, charts and tables. On both Apple and IBM systems there are freely available good open source alternatives to Microsoft's bought software, which may appeal to those on a tight budget. Google Docs and Sheets provide similar functionality and are easy to edit with several different users. There is more on this in Chapter Three on dissertations.

CASP tools

To help you make sense of all this information there are some free tools available online. CASP is the Critical Appraisal Skills Program (CASP, 2014). It provides some great free downloads of checklists. This set of eight **critical appraisal** tools are designed to be used when reading research, these include tools for:

- systematic reviews
- randomized controlled trials
- cohort studies
- case control studies
- economic evaluations
- diagnostic studies
- qualitative studies
- clinical prediction rule.

CASP may be of most use in a dissertation where you will need to use a variety of resources and be able to comment on the **validity** of the resources and why you have used them and where your research fits in.

Other similar checklists are available and we will discuss how to create checklists for creating your own research in Chapter Nine. This further information may help some people with understanding how best to use these checklists.

What is important with any information you find, you need to:

- interpret – in your own words to get a deeper understanding
- compare – the evidence to other work available in the field
- analyse – the evidence and the findings
- evaluate – whether this is the best work to support your argument.

The checklists in CASP will be best used when you reach the analyse/evaluate section of your review and you match the resource you are assessing to the CASP review and answer the questions it poses.

Which resource is best?

We are now learning in a world where one does not need to go to a physical library to access the books available there. Everything is on the internet – yes? The internet provides free and paid for academic resources. These can range from the online version of existing journals to internet-only sources that include e-books and articles. Many students now complete whole assignments without using a physical library – is this good, bad, or not an issue?

Which is best? Do you need to include at least one book in your references? Can all your references be online references? While each awarding body will have its own guidelines for their assignments here are some tips for how to use different resources.

Before you skip straight to finding out how to use Google for everything, please note this word of caution:

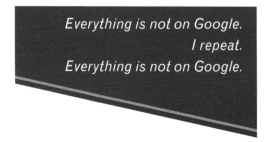

Everything is not on Google.
I repeat.
Everything is not on Google.

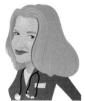

And I really mean that! While you can do a lot of research on the internet via standard search engines it does not mean you are accessing everything that is available. To show you have a full understanding of your subject area your tutor will expect to see a mix of resources. Starting with information from key textbooks, to evidence you have used e-books and journal articles that are not available on open access sites and that you have the skills to search databases to find appropriate information.

Understanding web addresses

You can tell a lot about a potential source by its URL. A URL is the 'address' or location of information on the internet. The proper name is uniform resource locator (URL) and the ending of URLs can tell you a lot about the website before you even look visit it.

.org   –   a not-for-profit organization **rscpca.org.uk**

.gov   –   government website, often accompanied by a country code, e.g. uk, **hmrc.gov.uk**

.ac   –   an academic institution, accompanied by the home country code of the institution, e.g. uk, **cam.ac.uk**

.nhs   –   large organizations may have their own URL **nhs.uk**

.uk   –   country codes to denote the home country: .ie = Ireland; .fr = France **veterinaryireland.ie**

.edu   –   used by US higher education institutions (colleges and universities) **harvard.edu**

.com   –   a company URL, can be used in any location **janervn.com**

.co.uk   –   a company URL for the UK **vetwholesaler.co.uk**

For academic research your searches may take you to a variety of these. Academic institutions will publish their own research, often in the form of working papers. Academic journals are usually run as a business venture, the majority by commercial publishers, some by research bodies and others by not-for-profit groups and charities. Paid access is via subscription or pay-per-article schemes. There is an increasing number of open access journals, where access to read is free. These usually are funded by author-paid publication fees, though some work on a wholly free to read, free to publish model.

A related source of research are conferences. Large conferences will often publish transactions of the paper presented, sometimes available freely, but often for a fee much like a journal.

Table 2.1 outlines the advantages and disadvantages of each type of common resource.

Table 2.1 Advantages and disadvantages of the most common resources

Resource	Advantage	Disadvantage	Examples/information
Books	Great starting point Provides general overview May be written in a less demanding style than academic papers	Infrequently updated Academic books may be peer reviewed May not be in depth enough for all your research	BSAVA manuals
Popular/industry magazines	Great starting point Written in an easy to access style Current issues/events discussed	Not peer reviewed May contain a mix of facts and opinion that may be hard to differentiate May not be in enough detail for academic work	*Veterinary Times* General news magazines that may cover veterinary issues
Journal articles	Aimed at researchers like you In depth on the subject area Full information on author, research methods, references Usually peer reviewed (but do check)	May require payment to access (may be accessible through your course provider)	*The Veterinary Nurse* *The Vet Record* *British Journal of Nursing* *Veterinary Nursing Journal*

Internet search engines	Easy to use Easy to access Can find a lot of information Good starting point for research and to familiarize yourself with the common terminology Can use to find support tools such as online dictionaries and referencing aids	No control over what it searches No quality control May be hard to find information on authors of work or establish when it was created Anyone can publish work Pages may not remain live and so may not be accessible for a tutor to check Copyright can be ambiguous (misconception that if it is on the web it is freely reusable) Results generated by popularity of website host as well as key words	Google, Bing
Library catalogues	Only published work listed All of an academic standard Grouped by subject and specialism Can search using age of information or number of citations Can get librarian help if needed	May only be available if you are a member of the library May need to learn some further database research skills	May overlap with online databases RCVS Knowledge University library British Library There are librarians to help you – never underestimate their skills
Online academic databases	Only published work stored All of an academic standard Grouped by subject and specialism Can search using age of information or number of citations	May need to learn some further online research skills If not accessing through a library or course provider may need to pay to see full article	May overlap with library catalogue Athens Abstracts Science Direct Web of Knowledge RCVS Knowledge

Visiting a library	Only published work stored	May not be one close to you	There are librarians to help you – never underestimate their skills
	All of an academic standard		
	Grouped by subject and specialism		
	Can search using age of information or number of citations		
	Can get librarian help if needed		
	Can be a good way to avoid distractions		

Using the library

Yes, you still need to use a library. It may not mean that you use the actual building that houses the books, instead many libraries now also provide amazing online resources. However, you should still know how to access the information in the building.

Libraries will store and access books using a classification system. There are several different types used, Dewey is the most common, which categorize books first by general subject area, then into further subject areas and then by alphabetical order by author's surname. This means you may need to find information from the veterinary section, life sciences, nursing or humanities.

Once you have located a work in the library catalogue it will give you a number, which guides you to where you will find the book in the library. It will guide you to the correct area, correct shelf and then you can work along the books and check the number and authors name until you find the correct book.

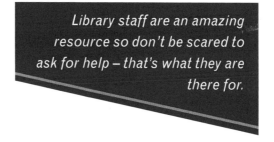

Library staff are an amazing resource so don't be scared to ask for help – that's what they are there for.

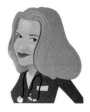

Some areas of the library will become familiar but as nursing research can cover many different fields you may be searching in new areas of the library or in new libraries. Each one will be laid out in a similar fashion and will have skilled researchers available to help you. I would advise visiting the library just to familiarize yourself with its layout and classification system. If the library runs study skills sessions then take advantage of them; they will reduce the time you spend researching and can provide you with better quality evidence, which can mean higher grades.

Types of research

Evidence-based resources can be divided by the type of research used to achieve results: **qualitative** and **quantitative**. In the veterinary nursing field, you will probably find many research papers use a mix of these and you will find your argument better supported by providing a range of research as evidence. Each type has its benefits and drawbacks and you will need to decide which type will provide the best support for your work.

Quantitative

Quantitative methods are used a lot in scientific research. Quantitative research is countable data. It shows changes that occur that can be accurately measured. In veterinary nursing this could be research to show if using bubble wrap to cover a patient during surgery reduces heat loss more than using a blanket. The results would show changes in temperature according to patient type, type of body wrap and length of surgery.

Much of our research may involve quantitative data as we routinely measure the patient journey and outcomes based on numerical data, for instance:

* temperature
* weight
* drug dose ranges administered
* blood parameters
* urinalysis parameters
* life expectancy.

This type of data is objective – it is a matter of fact rather than an opinion and while an author can give their opinion based on the results or the way research was carried out the data can only be presented as it was recorded.

Qualitative

Qualitative analysis of information is used when the information collected is not countable, or measurable using known scales, such as weight or time. It is used in nursing research in several ways.

First, it is used in research when the findings are discussed. This might include information on what other results we would expect to see from the patients or what these results could mean for the future. It is also used when we discuss outcomes, such as patient demeanor or their behavioral response to medication. While researchers can convert results into quantitative data by scoring behaviour on a scale, as in the commonly used pain score charts, we still need to describe how we arrive at grading this type of behavior.

Qualitative analysis would also be required if we researched the benefits of different coverings for cats during surgery. The quantitative research would show the numerical data and the qualitative would show discussions on the differences between different types of coverings, for example, wool blanket, fleece, bubble wrap. This can be a more subjective type of research where the author's opinions carry more weight than in quantitative research. There is not the numerical data to support or disprove a viewpoint.

Many research papers will carry an element of both types of data so being knowledgeable about how both are used will help you.

Primary and secondary evidence

Not all resources are presenting their own research. Many papers and even whole databases contain what is called secondary resources. You may be asked to specifically use evidence from primary resources rather than secondary resources. There are some important differences between the two.

Primary

An original publication with **primary** research data, that has been collected and analysed by the authors presenting it. The research may include results of questionnaires, observations and experiments. They are sometimes referred to as research articles.

Primary research is usually published by academic journals. This is still a growing area for veterinary nursing, but at present there is limited research data. Academic journals can be from any country and in veterinary nursing there are good publications from Australia and the USA:

- *The Veterinary Nurse* – peer reviewed
- *Veterinary Nursing Journal* – peer reviewed
- *Australian Veterinary Nurses Journal* – peer reviewed
- *Today's Veterinary Nurse* (formerly *Today's Veterinary Technician*) – USA, – free digital version available
- *NZ Vet Nurse Journal*

Secondary

Secondary resources cite or use other primary resources, and are published after the original source. Articles may not be on exactly the same topic area and there is always the possibility that the original material is used in a way the original author did not intend. If the original data is the area of interest for you it is best to source the original material, read and cite that.

Secondary resource databases include the Cochrane Library and NICE (National Institute for Health and Care Excellence), where new sources of information are gathered from reviews of primary sources.

The journals mentioned above will also contain secondary sources, as many vet nurses produce literature reviews on subject areas. Such articles can be a useful introduction to a range of primary sources, which you can then go on to read.

RCVS Knowledge is our industry' online database. It provides useful knowledge summaries of commonly asked questions. These summaries look at all the evidence available and put forward a summary about the quality of the evidence and whether there is enough evidence to make a decision for or against the proposed treatment plans.

Online database searching

There are now many online databases to search, some available online and some linked to a physical library. These require some different skills from using an open search engine such as Google.

Which database to use is the first decision. Your college or university will probably already have a preferred database that you are directed to when you log into their library. There are a large number of databases for academic work, and each has its benefits and drawbacks.

They are differentiated by the subject areas they cover, the type of data they hold and how they store and rate their information.

To make more sense of this we will consider three databases:

- CABAbstracts
- Jstor
- Pubmed.

All three have scientific data. Pubmed specializes in just medical data. CABAbstracts covers all applied life sciences and has a large veterinary section. Jstor focuses more on the humanities and social sciences, but it does have medicine and science sections, but no specific veterinary sub-section.

CABAbstracts is a full text resource that is used by the RCVS Knowledge database. This is available through membership of the RCVS Knowledge library or your college library and provides access to the main veterinary nursing journals and 97% of the veterinary research produced worldwide. Used in conjunction with databases, such as Pubmed, it can provide a comprehensive view of current veterinary research. Journal issues take around 3 months to appear in the database.

Jstor has a narrow selection of journals. Originally it was a collection of back issues, and so it has all issues from the start of the journal but may not have the most recent issues from the last 3–5 years. However, it is a full-text resource and is free once you have signed up.

Pubmed is likely to pop up even in your Google searches. It differs from the other two databases as it is an index only database. It holds information on huge amounts of free and paid for information.

Pubmed does not hold the full text.

It may have a link to get you to the full text and it has the information you need to decide if you wish to find the information. It displays the author details, publisher, the abstract and the number of citations.

There are many more databases. With all databases, you need to be aware that the time delay between writing and publishing sometimes as long as (18–24 months) means changes can have occurred that might make what you are writing obsolete. Therefore, I will not recommend any one database, but will give you the information to find the best path for you.

There is the option to search multiple databases at once. Your college or university database will most likely do this already so do check what you are searching when you log in to their system.

Currently the most comprehensive databases for us to use would be your college or university database, or a mixture of RCVS Knowledge, Pubmed and not forgetting Google as a starting point.

RCVS Knowledge is accessible in several ways:

- free access to the library for books and journals at Belgravia House for all RVNs
- low-cost access to the online catalogue
- free to join email alerts on veterinary nursing journal articles
- ability to order copies of articles for a set fee even if not a member.

Or you can join for around £50 a year and get access to all the information for free. This service is subsidized by the RCVS and is a great way to access appropriate research information once you have qualified and no longer have access to your college or university database.

Once you have decided on your database then you need to find out how best to search for the information you need. For free searches try Google, Pubmed and CABAstracts – CABi has a free trial for you to use. Jstor is useful for nursing subjects that cover the humanities rather than scientific information.

Types of search

While searching with key words is popular and is the most common way we use search engines in our daily lives there are better ways to search. Key words do not prioritize words or link them as a phrase. Therefore, if you searched with the words – veterinary nurse – you will be shown information that contains these two words, but not necessarily together. An article on an NHS nurse's visit to their local vets would show up but not have any mention of a 'veterinary nurse'.

To help reduce the amount of unrelated content there are other options. The database itself may have advanced search options (Figure 2.4). These let you select where they search for certain words in specific areas.

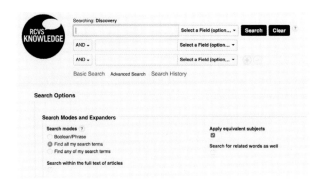

Figure 2.4 RCVS Knowledge search page. © RCVS Knowledge

RCVS Knowledge 2017

The drop-down choices offer you the options to search in three different areas choosing for each from:

- publication title
- article title
- author
- full text content
- abstract.

It also allows you to search for information on:

- any author affiliation
- key words
- any funding agencies
- reference list
- ISBN/ISSN – a book's or serial's (journal) unique reference number
- DOI – the unique reference number given to a digitally available resource (digital object identifier).

While it may take some more time to input this further information it reduces the amount of erroneous information you may get and also ensures you focus on what you are looking for. Before heading off to try this out, read a bit further and see what you can do with the words you put in each line – it might surprise you!

Boolean searches

Boolean searching is another option. By using 'and – or – not' between words it limits or expands your search.

AND, OR, NOT

If you wanted a wide initial search, then it is best to use OR. This would mean you search for 'diabetes cat OR dog', then information about either species would show.

If you use AND between words it looks for data with both these words in. Therefore, searching for information on pet diabetes you could look for 'diabetes cat AND dog' to include both. This will narrow your potential results as any articles that only focus on one species will not show on your search.

Finally, using NOT limits your search in a different way. If you had looked at both searches above and found there was significantly more written about feline diabetes than canine then searching for 'diabetes cat NOT dog' would remove all canine based resources.

Once you have established in more detail what you are searching for it is worth considering how much more detailed your questions could be. If you are searching for information on older cats and diabetes you are starting to add in several key words or phrases into your search. If you put in every possible variable it will take longer and it may narrow the return too much and not yield what you are looking for.

'Short cuts make long delays.' – J.R.R. Tolkien, The Fellowship of the Ring

Searching for 'phrases' and prioritising words

Another option is searching for a phrase. This lets you tell the search engine what you mean when you type in – veterinary nurse. If you type in – veterinary nurse – it searches as above, for those two words, together, apart, in any context. However, if you put "veterinary nurse" in double quotation marks it makes the search engine hunt for the words as a phrase. Meaning it will not find any articles on human nurses visiting the vets, unless they also mention veterinary nurses.

Advanced searching also has options to specify the order of words and to allow you to search for words with multiple endings in one easy way.

An example of search results via Google

If you were looking for information on kidney transplants in cats there are a few hurdles to getting the perfect search words. We know people use the words renal and kidney interchangeably. We also know there are variations on transplant. It could be described as transplantation, transplanted, transplanting. This could mean searching using six different phrases. There is an easier way.

By adding *, sometimes called a wildcard, to the end of a word you 'truncate' it. Meaning you shorten it to the important root part of the word and tell the search engine you are happy to see the word with any possible ending.

You can also advise the search engine on the importance of words in your search. If you put in kidney, renal, transplant and cats it will weigh these four equally. This can mean you could get information on kidney diets for cats, or other treatments to avoid transplants. Which may not be what you were looking for. You can use brackets to tell the search engine which words are most important.

Putting it all together

Advanced search strategies can be used together. You can truncate words, use Boolean terms and prioritize words and phrases all at once. This will take some practice. You can use these options on Google so before you head over to more advanced databases see what a difference some planning of your search terms can do.

I searched for information on renal transplants in cats on Google using two different options. The first was using standard key words – renal transplants in cats. It yielded a number of hits, but the top ones were from general news resources (Figure 2.5). Not really appropriate for an academic search.

Figure 2.5 Standard Google search results

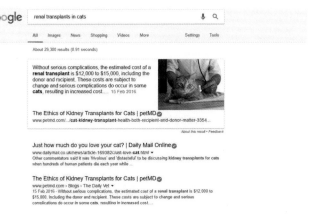

I then searched using – transplant* and (renal kidney) in cats. A combination of Boolean and advanced searches. The results are shown in Figure 2.6.

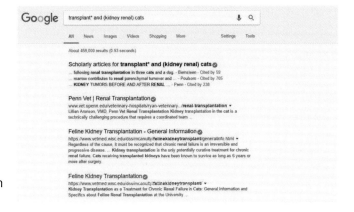

Figure 2.6 Boolean search results from Google

Nearly 500,000 hits and the list starts with scholarly articles and includes information from many educational institutions, a much better result for academic research.

With thanks to the team at RCVS Knowledge for all their help.

Further research options

There is yet another option. It takes more time to consider but it would be useful for more in-depth work, such as a dissertation, or for when you need concise information on a set area, such as when you write SOPs or evidence protocols at work.

It helps to break up the search into smaller pieces. This can be done methodically by using PICO (Northedge, 2005).

Patient/population – who is affected?
Intervention   – what is the treatment?
Comparisons   – what can this be compared to?
Outcomes   – what happens to the patients?

This takes your one search for information on diabetic older cats and makes you focus on what you are looking for. As an example, if you are interested in finding any information on treating diabetic cats with medication that does not require injections – as you have encountered many clients who do not like the concept of injecting their cat daily and do not feel able to do this – how do you find the information that gives helpful information?

Table 2.2 PICO table

Search areas	What you are looking for	Terms, acronyms, US/UK spellings
P	Cats 8+ years old in UK	Cat, cats, feline, felines, aged, geriatric, older, senior, UK, GB, Britain, England, Scotland, Wales, Northern Ireland
I	Non-injectable (tablet) medication for diabetes	Tablets, pills, oral, parenteral, prescription
C	Diet, weight, injection treatment, other non-injection treatment	Food, nutrition, diet, fibre, protein, prescribed, insulin, injection, USA, Australia
O	Diabetic stability, QOL, rehomed and life expectancy	Stable, hypoglycaemia, hyperglycaemia, nadir, glucose curve, monitoring, urinalysis, dip stick, euthanasia, quality of life, QOL, end stage, fructosamine, lab samples, testing, ear samples, home testing, concurrent disease, mmols

Keeping track of your research

Researching efficiently is an amazing skill. It takes time to get right and it is time well spent. But it also means you need to be good at the more boring side of academic work. The labelling, filing and general tidiness that means you can find lecture notes, reading lists and research notes at a later date. It may be worth checking out the information in Chapter One again on note making and filing information.

It is good practice to keep several documents open while you research. This could be in Word format as one of the documents makes a great start for your reference list for later.

How to start your reference list

First, you need a list of all the websites you have visited from which you took information. At the start of your research you may not know which bits of information you find you will use in your work. I have found that some interesting information I thought was peripheral to my search at the start actually becomes very important later on. I have learnt the hard way the importance of keeping a full record of all the information accessed – so you don't need to! You will also need this extra information if you are required to sit an oral exam based on work you have submitted. We will cover this in more detail in Chapter Six. It is also a good way to see how much more efficient you have become as a researcher. The list of information accessed but not used will become smaller.

A 'full record' includes the URL, the title of the books/articles/webpages you have read and where the information was in the document – chapters and page numbers. As well as the URL, make a list of where you accessed them and what restrictions there were. Some text books require that you order them in advance. Some cannot be removed from the library so you need to factor in time to work in the library. These are pieces of information you are likely to forget while you are researching but may be needed in a hurry if you want to check a quote or piece of information.

For larger assignments, you may find it easier to keep direct quotes in a separate document that you write or type, on the potential direct quotes from the books or you may wish to combine all the information into one place – do this using colours and fonts to differentiate quotes, summaries or different types of resource.

Make sure the list of websites contains the URL you accessed it from and the title of the page you were reading. To make it easier in the future to create a reference list include all the information you will need later on now, so you do not waste time later going back to find it.

- Author name(s)
- Year of publication
- Title of article or chapter
- Journal or book title
- Publisher
- Location of publication
- Volume/issue/page number for journals
- URL/DOI of online articles and date accessed

It does not have to be in the correct format or even have the information in the correct order.

It is easy to copy and paste these. It also helps to include a brief reason why the page or document was of interest to you and the location of the information. Some documents you find can be large and there is little point in finding a great quote on page 87 of a 200-page document if you do not note this down and then cannot remember which page it was on when you need to check the exact wording.

Quotes and potential citations

If you are reading information online there is another document it is worth creating, as you read you will find pieces of information that really interest you. Keep a document with the article title at the top and then copy and paste potential quotes onto this document. This is a separate document from your initial list of URLs. Think of the list of URLs as the start of your reference list and this list as the start of your compilation of quotes.

If you are used to hand writing notes it can be hard to move to using a computer or tablet. But once it comes to collating all you have read, having everything in a single format that you can easily copy and paste is easier and time saving. It is worth looking at write to text software which allows you to write on a device, which then saves your hand-written notes as typed text.

For all potential quotes or citations record the page number you found them on too. It is much quicker to use this document in the future when writing your work instead of having to look up individual pieces of information again.

While it may feel like a lot of extra work it really is essential to keep a record of your work as you do it. It will save you time later and will provide evidence of where you have reached with your research each time you go back to it.

> 'Where did you go to, if I may ask?' said Thorin to Gandalf as they rode along. 'To look ahead,' said he. 'And what brought you back in the nick of time?' 'Looking behind,' said he."
> – J.R.R. Tolkien, The Hobbit

Keeping your research safe

As so much of your work is going to be researched, written, edited and submitted via computers and the internet it is worth taking some time to think about how you will store and retrieve this information.

As I have already mentioned you need to be good at labelling, naming and filing. You can have your own system and no one else needs to know about it if you do not want them to, but ensure it is systematic and works for you.

However, you need to use systems already available for saving and storing work. It can be the biggest hurdle in academic work. Saving and having copies of up-to-date work in case of system error or hard drive failure or worse is so important. Most universities will have a clause in the submission of work that states computer failure is not a reason for an extension or not to submit! See Chapter One on suggestions for how to store files.

> Therefore, take pride in your work and cherish and save it.

Research for exams

Research for exams may be undertaken using these research skills. However, you will find that as exams are a timed and focused assessment of your knowledge they do not require the same depth of understanding as an assignment. The examiners will be looking more for extended knowledge based on course notes, lectures and the course reading list.

This does not mean you can ignore your new-found skills, you can still use them but your study path will be slightly different. Chapters Four to Seven deal with succeeding in various types of exams. But first let's head to Chapter three to see how to write about all the information we have found.

> *'It's the job that's never started as takes longest to finish.'*
> *– J.R.R. Tolkien,* The Fellowship of the Ring

 Review Chapter 2 and how to apply what you have learned with the Reflective Template.

Chapter 2 glossary

boolean – a way to use search engines

citations – providing a direct and clear reference back to another's work to indicate you have relied on it and to guide a reader to the resource

critical appraisal – similar to critical thinking, systematically assessing resources to ensure they are worth using

critical thinking – the skill of assessing information and documents that you may find and decide if they are valid resources

digital literacy – the ability to find appropriate information and assess its authenticity

eDatabase – electronic collection of information provided in a variety of formats

journal – academic publication, usually peer reviewed

medium – books, journals, conference proceedings, ebooks, ejournals, web pages, web sites peer review – articles that have been reviewed by industry/field peers before publication

primary (source) – original piece of research

provenance – the record of ownership of an academic resource

qualitative – research that involves things that are hard to measure

quantitative – research that involves measureable quantities – times, dates, amounts

reference – another's work you wish to note, you provide a citation in the text to the reference in the bibliography

resource – a medium that provides information to help your understanding of a subject

search engine – tool that allows you to search the internet (for example, Google)

secondary (source) – research that reports on, collects or reuses other resources, primary or secondary

validity – a resource that is factually sound

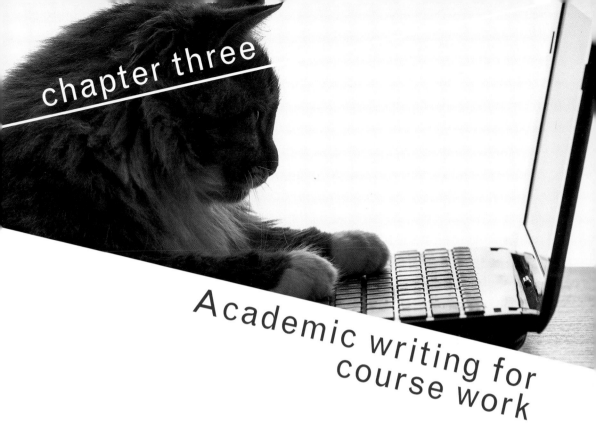

chapter three

Academic writing for course work

What is academic writing?

Academic writing is a key part of most courses. It is another skill that you will need to learn – but do not be put off, it is an achievable skill and gets better with practice.

You will not be expected to be a proficient academic writer at the start of your course, and part of the assessment criteria will be about giving you **feedback** which you can use to improve. In particular, scientific academic writing is a very concise way of presenting your **research** or data. It was more presentation conventions than fiction or writing for arts or humanities courses. These conventions will help you to present your data and the knowledge you have gained in a clear manner. It is important that you use your own words, as this shows a deeper understanding of a subject than just stringing together a number of quotes from the writing of others and it also ensures you do not **plagiarize** work, your own or

> *'Much to learn you still have'*
> – *Yoda*, Star Wars: Episode II –
> Attack of the Clones

others – even if you did not intend to. Coming from an arts background with a history degree I struggled to meet the demands of scientific academic writing, but I persevered!

The way you set out your work will also allow for more helpful feedback from your tutors. This is especially important at the start of your course. The feedback can be on the references you cite, the style of writing or the mechanics of writing – spelling errors and other issues that detract from the point you are making. If it is clear what you are saying and why you are using the evidence you have, then it is easier for tutors to give feedback and provide you with help for the future.

The challenges of academic writing include:

• what to say – information and ideas
• how to say it – style as well as substance
• engaging your audience.

It can help to think about your work as if you were writing for publication. This is the type of standard that tutors are looking for. You can also use the writing styles of articles you have researched and liked as a basis for approaching how to present your work.

Planning your writing

If you can imagine the process of producing an assignment is similar in structure to a well filled sandwich (Figure 3.1). The researching at the start and editing at the end are the slices of bread. Thin, supportive, but not the main event. You do not spend that long considering the bread, or considering the beginning and end of the writing process. The important part, the most time consuming and interesting part is the filling – the writing, surely? Well, no, not really.

Each part of your assignment is important but may take a different amount of time, so be prepared to alter your initial plans if you assumed the writing would take the longest amount of time. The writing can be the shorter part of the process as the research and editing can take more time than you had planned.

If you research well and use active reading (see Chapter Two) and make notes as you go (see Chapter One) then you will have in fact have already

The sandwich is less this

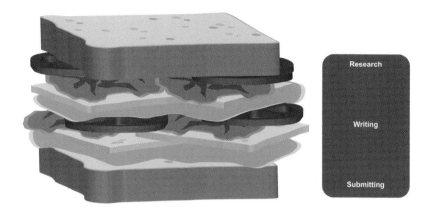

and more this

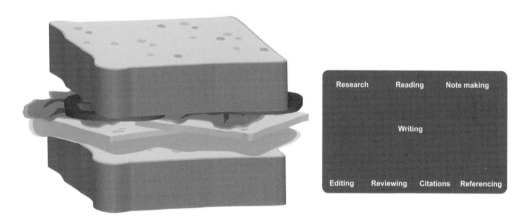

Figure 3.1 The academic writing sandwich (artist: Jorgen Mcleman)

started the writing part and may actually find it easier and quicker than you imagined. Depending on the marking criteria for your course you may get a substantial amount of marks for referencing and **citation**, similar to that for content, and so you should spend time to make sure these are correct and match the style of referencing you have been asked to use. Check the marking criteria at the outset and use it to guide the split of your effort on the assignment. There is little point spending three-quarters of your time on an element that only gets one-quarter of the marks.

How do I get started?

Writing is about sitting down and producing words. J.K. Rowling may have produced modern masterpieces sitting in a café all day but very few people have the level of drive and concentration to achieve academic level work in a noisy environment.

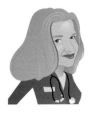

It isn't angst-ridden wanderings around parks waiting for 'inspiration'

If you are struggling to write, then make it easy on yourself. Consider the part you are stuck on and just write down what you know, or your ideas about that area for 5 minutes – make sure you time yourself. Stop when the timer goes off and review what you have written. (Timers for smartphones and tablets are available in the online resources.) Try to read it as a pair of 'new eyes' would and see where there are gaps in your knowledge and whether you have raised any questions that need to be answered. This common writing exercise can help you process information quickly and show you where there are gaps to be filled, questions to be researched and will hopefully show you that your ideas are coming together.

As with any academic work you will have deadlines and a limited time for each assessment. You will need to make decisions about how much time you have to spend on an assignment and also how much time you are able to give to each assessment, taking into account other assessments you may have deadlines for.

Northedge (2005) has a great checklist for planning assignments (Table 3.1). The first three steps are really important, take the time to consider them properly. It can seem that you need to research and head to Step 4 before deciding Steps 1–3 but it is crucial to know how much time you have and are able to spend on the assignment as well as ensuring you have checked what it is asking of you and that you are clear what they are looking for.

Table 3.1 Checklist for planning assignments (adapted from Northedge, 2005)

Step	Starting point	What you need to do	Tips
1	Decide how much time you have and how well you want to do	Aim for higher than passing to give leeway	Consider the assignment's effect on your overall grade – what does it count towards?
2	Plan your timetable	Set out diary with work, college, family and leisure time	Be honest! Your leisure time may need to reduce Try to get help with family responsibilities if you can Are you working efficiently? Using online resources instead of travelling to the library? Not looking at Facebook when you are meant to be working!
3	Check the assignment title and what questions you are expected to answer Make sure you understand the questions	Can you identify which part of the syllabus is covered and are there any reading lists or resources that can help you?	Check marking criteria, especially for referencing and citation information
4	Structure of answer	Make bullet points and notes on ideas of subjects to cover, arguments that might crop up	Consider the introduction and conclusion and how you will present the information
5	Research using course notes, references and reading lists	Use the information in Step 3 to start your research • start active reading and note making • keep records of research read and start reference list	Use your research skills to go beyond the resources provided and find further evidence to support your work
6	Write a first draft in your own words with references	Using Step 4 flesh out your bullet points into paragraphs and a first draft	As you write you can edit – you may need to move sections around as you form your arguments more fully
7	Edit spelling, grammar and style	Check, check and check again! Spell check, proofread, get a friend or colleague who you know is keen on good spelling to proofread **Read the work aloud as you go to make sure it makes sense!**	Be honest with yourself when editing and ask for advice if you are not sure. Becoming confident in your own editing will take time, so take it in little steps

Table 3.1 continued

Step	Starting point	What you need to do	Tips
8	Strengths weaknesses and layout	Are there any areas to improve? Does the finished piece still answer the assignment question AND meet the marking criteria?	Use the marking criteria as a checklist and make sure it is all covered
9	Edit and finalize referencing	Ensure you have used the referencing style requested	Do not rush this section. You may lose vital marks for poorly presented work and incorrect citations. Both are easy marks to gain after all your research
10	Submit on time and in appropriate place	Make sure you have more than one copy stored. Upload to the required website, or submit a hard copy well in advance	If the deadline is 9 p.m. on a Sunday are there people to help you if there is a website issue? If your wifi stops working what are your other options – coffee shop wifi might not let you upload large documents. Be prepared! For paper copies have it delivered by hand, or posted via recorded delivery. Whichever method, get a receipt to prove time and place of submission – if the work is lost then you can prove it is not because you did not submit

To make a start you need access to all the information on the module the assignment is for and to consider how it affects your overall grade. Some modules may be weighted so they carry more marks towards your final mark. While you never want to do badly in any assessment, there are some that may matter more and you should check and judge your effort.

> 'Do or do not; there is no try'
> – Yoda, Star Wars: Episode V – The Empire Strikes Back

For academic writing, there are a few rules to follow.

- Do not use shortened/contracted versions of words:

    - don't – do not
    - shouldn't – should not.

- Present numbers according to the style required. A common style is to write in full numbers one–ten and then to write in figures from 11 onwards.
- If you are using acronyms write them in full on first use followed by the acronym in parentheses after, then use the acronym: Royal College of Veterinary Surgeons (RCVS).
- For **punctuation** and citation use the same style thorough the assignment. Do not change part of the way through.

Your course provider may have some more guidelines so check these as part of your planning and again when editing.

Spelling, punctuation, grammar

I have mentioned this above but it really cannot be overstated that being perfect in all three of these areas is essential. If you are not confident with spelling, punctuation and **grammar**, then do not worry when you are researching and starting your work. These can all be perfected in the editing process.

Why is it important? Poor presentation of work will make it harder for the reader to understand your argument and see the important parts of your work – your thinking and reasoning. Spelling, grammar and punctuation provide the framework in which you present your research and ideas: done well they go unnoticed and your research shines through; done badly and it can be all the reader will take away, as they cannot access your research.

Correct spelling and producing work that can be read easily is important in creating that professional image. But do not let that hold you back from getting words on the page.

> It is important when presenting your work to create a professional image.

Correcting these things can all be done once you have completed putting your ideas on paper. As long as you can understand your work as you write it, you can tidy it up later, but make sure to leave enough time to do this, it can take longer than you think.

Make sure your computer is set to 'English – UK' for spell checker if in the UK. They often default to US English. If not then your spell checker will note as errors words that are spelled correctly for a UK audience. Spell checkers are very useful, but they are limited, come of the things the spell checker will not alert you to include:

- similar words with different meanings – there/their
- incorrect use of its/it's
- names incorrectly spelt – especially important for citation
- technical terms the dictionary does not know
- incorrect numbers, for example, dates
- repetition of **sentences** or **paragraphs** – so be careful copying and pasting.

You can add names and technical terms to your online dictionary so your spell checker learns to recognize them – but make sure your entry is exactly as you want it, and you include any variations of the word that are similar that may be altered by spell checker, to prevent future issues.

Punctuation can be a minefield. There are so many rules to follow, yet poor punctuation can have a big impact on how easy your writing is to understand.

This example shows how a comma can help:

Most of the time, travellers worry about their luggage.

Now remove the comma after the fourth word to totally change the meaning of this sentence:

Most of the time travellers worry about their luggage.

Without the comma 'time travellers' are linked as the same subject. The comma separates them and allows a sentence to make two points – that travellers worry about luggage and that this is a common occurrence. Without the comma, you would need two sentences to make the same point.

Commas are used for lists, to separate out the items on a list – but not before the final item is added with an 'and' at the end.

Unneutered dogs may suffer from pyometras, testicular cancers, prostate problems and behavioural issues.

They are also used to join sentences where you are using conjunctions, such as 'but' or 'and' to join them. You may recall being told never to start a sentence with 'But'? The comma is the punctuation to save you from this issue.

The vet wanted to spey the dog next week, but the owner was not able to make the appointment.

This flows better than two sentences and still shares all the relevant information.
Where there is 'extra information' in a sentence, a pair of commas are used to demonstrate this. The idea is that the sentence should stand alone without the extra information.

The owner, who was parked on a double yellow line, wished to settle the bill quickly.

There are other rules for commas but as they are rarely used in scientific writing I have not explained them here. I think there is quite enough for you to focus on for now, and as I said before, you can correct your punctuation once you have the words and ideas written down.
Apostrophes can also cause problems as they are used in several ways: -

- to show possession – Jim's dog
- to show an omission – it is becomes it's.

They are never used for plurals: The dogs are in the field. Or when there is a possessive adjective: The dog ate its bone.
As with all writing there are different styles and ways of using punctuation. Keep to a style you are confident using throughout the assignment and stick to it. It is worth checking with your university if they recommend any particular styles.
The world of punctuation is an interesting one. I could write a whole book just on punctuation for academic writing. If you are interested in punctuation

in general then I can recommend reading Lynne Truss' (2009) amazing book, *Eats, Shoots & Leaves.*

Sentences, paragraphs, syntax

This may seem obvious, but do you use sentences properly? We often write as if we were speaking to someone else but in academic writing this will not be appropriate. We need to produce formal written work and make what we are saying very clear and concise.

A sentence starts with a capital letter and ends with a full stop. It should contain a subject and a verb, meaning it should be able to convey information about the subject matter and what it is doing. This makes it sound more complicated than it is.

What it means to you and I is that a sentence needs to make sense! And that can be harder than it sounds. It needs to ensure it will read the same way to all readers of the text and does rely on the further information we get from seeing or hearing people speak to make sense.

We often talk in incomplete sentences as we can demonstrate further knowledge with gestures, intonation of voice and body language.

One tip is to keep sentences short. This means it is easier for the reader to focus on the meaning. If this starts to produce work that is hard to read as it lacks a flow, use commas and joining words (conjunctions) to put sentences together. The meaning of your work will remain clear but the speed of writing will not be diminished.

While we are making notes and writing down ideas we may not think about sentence structure. Once you are heading to your first draft you need to make sure the sentences are clearly stating what you want to say. Where you have several points to make, you need to carefully consider which are the most important and that there is a logical flow. This is where good use of punctuation can help. There may be another way to present what you want to say, you should consider this.

Paragraphs are then built from groups of sentences. A paragraph should contain information on one subject area, but it can contain different viewpoints about the subject area. In some ways it is like a mini-essay on its own. You need an introductory sentence, then further information and a conclusion sentence. Here is an example from an article I wrote.

> **Uniforms should be laundered at 60 degrees on the same day as the shift.** They should also be tumble dried as this provides a second heat source to kill bacteria (Riley 2015). Uniforms should be laundered only with other uniforms but not scrub suits. Scrubs suits should be laundered at 71 degrees. Riley (2015) states standard detergents available to the public are suitable for washing uniforms if the correct amounts are used and the temperature and cycle length adhered to. **The author would recommend further research in the use of veterinary detergents and virucidal agents for uniforms used in isolation facilities as there is little current information.**

The emboldened sentences are the introduction and conclusion. The paragraph is introduced as being about laundry temperatures for uniforms. Further information is included on types of uniform and temperatures required for each type. The conclusion sentence covers the fact there is little information on laundry detergents, which would normally have been discussed as part of the laundry process. However, there is not enough research relevant to the topic to discuss it in an academic article.

Although this is not a perfect example of a paragraph it gives you an idea of how one is formed. This example gives you a mini-essay on one part of a larger subject area. You can understand the points made and it adds to the overall understanding of the information in the article.

Syntax is a subject we do not often think about yet we are very aware of it. Some sentences can look strange and although still understand them it is takes a little more work than it should.

Syntax is well illustrated by the film character – Yoda. In English, we usually construct sentences as subject – verb – object. Meaning we put our sentences together like this:

Yoda grasped the lightsaber.

Where Yoda is the subject, the verb is 'grasped' and the lightsaber is the object. However, Yoda would say:

Grasped Yoda the lightsaber.

He would still put the emphasis on the second word as we would, giving the unusual intonation to his speaking. This is because Yoda puts the verb at the start of the sentence, then the subject (himself), then the object. While this seems unusual to English speakers there are some languages that use this type of structure, for example Hawaiian. While it is not the way an English speaker would normally construct sentences, it is not totally alien, even if Yoda is a little alien!

This is just to emphasize the importance of setting out your information in a way that makes sense, especially if you are using new words and terminology that you are unsure about.

An example of poor sentence structure:

Before discussing the advantages of prescription diets in felines, it is important to understand the disadvantages to be found in the treatment of many diseases by medication alone.

The problem lies in the use of 'it'. There is no clear subject to the sentence, it is not clear what 'it' refers back to. This could be more clearly presented:

Before discussing the advantages of prescription diets in felines, we need to understand the disadvantages to be found in the treatment of many diseases by medication alone.

Or:

To fully understand the advantages of prescription diets in treating feline diseases we should consider the evidence when treating by medication alone.

As with all writing, editing, reading aloud and asking others to proofread will help you ensure you are writing work that is well presented and easy to read. As you write more your skills will improve, I promise.

> 'In a dark place we find ourselves, and a little knowledge lights our way.'
> – Yoda, Star Wars: Episode III – Revenge of the Sith

Academic writing – putting it all together

The building blocks of writing (spelling, grammar, punctuation, sentences and paragraphs) can be altered once you have your ideas and arguments decided. As you create your content you will need to consider the style of writing. For scientific academic writing there are a few guidelines to bear in mind.

- Scientific – use correct terminology and ideas, present research and debates with regard to theories and theoretical perspectives – that is, lab results over evidence-based veterinary medicine (EBVM.)
- Minimal waffle – word counts are tight and you need to use them well.
- Professional – show data, case studies and real-life situations EBVM.

You may want to consider emulating the style of some journals or writers who you have enjoyed reading. To be clear this is copying the way in which they write and present information, *not* the content. We will cover plagiarism later, for now, consider the different styles of academic writing:

- arts essays
- scientific essays
- reports
- case studies
- assignments.

You will not get academic writing perfect at the first attempt, it takes time and practice. That is why the more heavily weighted, or higher academic levels of work are usually found towards the end of your course. You will have had feedback about your writing from previous assignments and can should apply this to improve your work.

I cover more on feedback in the chapter on work-based learning (Chapter Eight), but with every bit of feedback, do make sure you read it, understand it and ask questions of the tutors if you are unclear, so you can make the best use of it to improve your work.

Who is this third person?

Writing in the **third person**. This is expected in most professional and academic titles, but what does it mean, who are they and where did they come from?

First person

As in the writing of this book I am writing from my perspective and so I use 'I', 'we' and 'my', which are all personal pronouns.

Second person

This is one step removed from first person writing and uses 'you', 'your' and 'yours' as pronouns. I refer to the prospective readers as 'you' as I cannot write from your perspective but I am writing for your needs.

Third person

As in the example above on laundering uniforms, the third person uses 'they' and if referring to individuals would use 'he' or 'she'. Some colleges, universities or publications have their own preferred presentation style so please check that you will meet the assessment or publishing criteria before you start writing.

The third person is a formal way of writing and removes personal bias, which is important in academic writing. It gives a sense of objectivity, especially when combined with the passive tense. Reading writing in the third person, you will see constructions such as 'The researcher(s)/author(s) recorded . . .'.

Plagiarism – is this all your own work?

We also need to consider a very serious aspect of academic writing: plagiarism. To quote Boyd (2014: 102):

> Plagiarism is 'Using someone else's work and ideas without acknowledging them properly. Either direct quotes using " " or paraphrasing others. Or using your own work twice.'

If I copied and pasted the sentence above into another chapter, but did not state it was from an author called Boyd, it would be using the work without acknowledging who produced it, even though I have referenced it here. It is important to follow the style of referencing your college asks you to use. There is more on this later in this chapter and you can always get more information on the chosen style from your college or university. You will also note there are times where I have referenced my own writing in these chapters – again it is necessary to say that even if I have written something it is not original writing for this assessment or topic and so I need to acknowledge the source.

The previous chapters have set you on the right road to avoiding plagiarism. By keeping organized notes on your reading and research you have already started making a reference list. This will help you allocate notes and comments made about your reading.

When I make notes, because I have such bad handwriting I type my research notes, I have direct quotes in normal font with ' ' around the words. Indirect quotes in normal font with NO ' ', and my thoughts and ideas in *italics*. For handwritten notes, you could use different coloured pens or use both sides of a note book – the right-hand page for quotes and the left-hand page for your own thoughts and ideas. This provides easy to read notes and this is essential when you look back at your research. It makes it clear what are your words and what are someone else's, avoiding accidental plagiarism.

Why is plagiarism such a serious issue? Put bluntly it is a form of cheating. Using someone else's work and presenting it as your own is cheating. It is the same as copying answers in an exam.

The majority of work you do will be submitted electronically. As you do this you are asked to confirm that this is all your own work – and then the work is often put through a software programme to show up any possible phrases or parts of scripts that match other work. This will also include other students' work from previous or current years. Copying a script from last year from the same module will be spotted. When you go on to publish, your work will be subjected to the same process by academic journals and book publishers.

Even if not spotted it is unlikely to lead to high marks as it is what you do with your research that matters. It is your opinions and ideas that matter and it is hard to match other people's writing and ideas exactly to your own and make it read well and make sense.

Proven plagiarism may lead to suspension or expulsion as it is such a serious issue. If you are struggling to produce work then ask for help, do not plagiarize. If you think you have accidentally plagiarized then check your notes and the texts used. Run the phrase or sentence through Google/database – if you have kept an accurate record then you should be able to find out where to search.

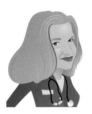

> *Finally, if in doubt about using a sentence or phrase that you can't identify as yours, or someone else's, follow the parachutist's safety mantra – if in doubt take it out!*

Structuring your writing

Your assignments will all follow a similar structure and it is worth taking time at the start of your course to establish how you will structure assignments. If you create a template of how to present information it will make it easier in the future.

Like any good story you will need a beginning, a middle and an end (Figure 3.2). This is essential as you need to communicate clearly with your reader what you are writing about, why you are writing about it, what you found out about it and what conclusions you have drawn.

Having a plan for where all the information from your research will be used in your assignment is really helpful and as you read around the subject certain things become clear, including:

- common themes in the field
- areas where more research is needed
- common viewpoints from known authors.

These will help you develop your viewpoint and will also guide you to the areas you will need to discuss in detail. While a good, clear introduction helps set up an assignment and make it easier to write and to read, you may find the

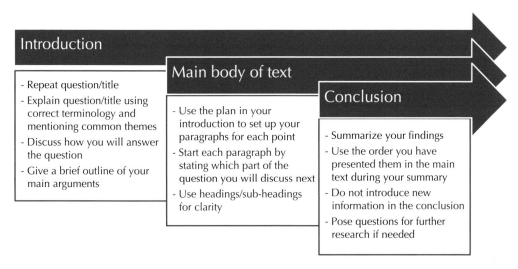

Figure 3.2 Structure for academic writing

introduction in full comes after you have fleshed out some paragraphs of the main body, clarifying your thoughts on all you have read. While you need to present your work in a logical fashion you may find you need to explore what you are saying in the assignment rather than writing an amazing introduction which makes statements you do not follow up. One strategy is to start with a rough introduction, but then to go back and refine it after you have written the main body. You can then check that you are not doing this.

You also want to make sure that your work meets the requirements from the marking criteria. While this will not cover what you need to include as content it will guide you on your writing and presentation skills. The marking criteria may well be looking for your use of language – is it appropriate at this level, do you use correct terminology confidently and avoid slang terms? It may include marks for spelling, grammar and punctuation. It may include marks for presenting a logical and well-balanced argument and for appropriate use of references and citations. What this means is that you need to ensure you have references that fulfil the criteria we mention later in this chapter and that you do not over use one reference or even one author to support your argument.

This can be very hard, especially once you start looking at choosing your own title and subject areas, such as for a **dissertation**. If there is little research it can be hard to meet these criteria and gain high marks.

Your dissertation

This is the 'ultimate' undergraduate assignment and it is a good time to talk about writing for your dissertation and the skills you will use that have been perfected through your assignment writing during your course.

This is probably the biggest piece of written work the majority of us will undertake. Dissertations vary from 7–10,000 words in length and are on a subject of your choosing. You may have the option to do a research project and focus your dissertation on this. Dissertations can be a literature review or involve you designing a research project to produce original data. Most dissertations that require original data will also need you to demonstrate the need for the data you collected, by first carrying out a short literature review of the subject area to highlight an area that needs more work.

While all the advice on writing assignments can be applied to writing your dissertation, you do need to think about how you choose what you write about. This time you are posing the question you wish to answer instead of answering a pre-set question.

While this may sound easier there are a few things to consider.

- What are your interests? This is a big task and you are likely to be more committed to a subject that interests and excites you.
- Will it be useful in the field of vet nursing today – for example, use of thiopentone in dogs is likely to be an outdated subject.
- Is there information already to support your topic, or can you demonstrate a gap in evidence that shows your research is valid.
- Who is your supervisor and what is their subject area(s).
- What are the ethical and financial implications of your proposed research.
- Will you have access to the cases, species, equipment you will need to do it properly?

As the profession progresses there is more vet nursing based research and evidence available. This is leading to a wider range of topics that can be covered, which is great news. However, it is likely you will need to include veterinary and relevant human care information to provide support for your ideas.

When deciding if a subject area or topic is right for you then you do need to consider:

- what information is available in this area
- whether it is well researched
- what can you bring that is new.

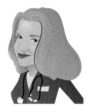

> *As you go through ideas it's advisable to start large and end up small!*

Start with a whole subject area and narrow down your list using the above considerations as filters as well as considering how broad your subject area is – try to refine your question area. It is very easy to start trying to answer too general a question and end up trying to cover too many bases and not providing enough focused analysis on any one thing.

You can further refine your question by considering personal factors, such as the type of practice you work in, personal interest or something that is happening in your local area. In the UK, we have seen an increase in cases of Seasonal Canine Illness (Alabama Rot), which require intensive nursing. There are many regional parasites that create complex nursing cases and may be of interest but as of yet have not been written.

You are likely to need to produce original research for your dissertation and with this comes the need to analyse the data you have produced. Before you worry about your maths skills there are numerous software packages that can do the hard maths for you. You just need to find a way to create meaningful data, decide how best to analyse it and then write about it. Easy really!

> *'If you end your training now – if you choose the quick and easy path as Vader did – you will become an agent of evil.'*
> *– Yoda, Star Wars: Episode V – The Empire Strikes Back*

Before we move on, I would like to provide a little terminology list – when you are reading about research and data you will need to use terms that may be new to you.

Dissertation terminology

Abstract – this is like an advert for your work. A short description of what you did, what happened and what you found out. They are very useful for people searching for your work so remember to include key words that people may use in a database search. You may not need one for academic submissions but they are interesting to write as they are a summary of your work and you can see more easily if you answer the question you set out to do.

Data – facts and figures from your research.

Ethics committee – if your research requires you to alter the way a patient is cared for to get data then you will need to get the approval of the college's ethics committee. This usually involves you completing an application process for the ethics committee where you outline the methods of your research and what they involve. At this stage, you will need to have confirmed where you are accessing patients or clients and have the consent of the veterinary establishment concerned. It is best to have written consent from the practice owner and those who will be involved in either helping you directly or recording data when you are not there.

Hypothesis – this is where you say what you think you will find out. If you are considering heat loss for surgical patients you may wish to narrow that by looking at the heat loss between admission and administration of a pre-med or between pre-med and induction. You may think that the heat loss between pre-med and induction is relevant to final post-op temperature and your hypothesis would state that. It is not important that you are right, that your hypothesis is correct, but that you test it. You are looking for information that would either provide evidence to support this statement or provide evidence to disprove it, that is, the heat loss between admission and pre-med was of more significance.

Metadata – data about data – this will all become clear when you start to collate the information gathered but it essentially means the structure and context of your data and is usually of greater interest to others once your research is complete and published.

Methodology – this sounds dramatic but it's describing the activities you will undertake to create research data – and we head back to your search for qualitative data or quantitative data or is it a mix of both?

Mixed methods – most research needs to be a mix of both types of research, and vet nursing is no different. In fact, vet nursing is often the perfect mix of numerical data and behavioural information.

Qualitative – data that is not numerical but shows opinions or behaviours. If you were researching the feeding of cats in a multi-cat household you would be finding out the food brands used, who fed them, the types and locations of the food bowls. Essentially the 'qualities' or descriptive data of what you are researching.

Quantitative – numerical data, so if using the example above of finding out about feeding in a multi-cat household you would find out numbers of cats, amounts of food purchased, amount consumed, times fed. Essentially numerical 'quantity' data of what you are researching.

Representativeness – how diverse is your group of subjects? If you are looking at research into a single species you should still be able to demonstrate a range of breeds, gender and age, as well as diverse ownership and information collated over a reasonable period of time.

Research – more than just finding the right information this time – original research – creating new information and ideas with an evidence base specifically designed by you.

Sample size – the number of subjects represented by your data.

Subject – a person, or animal in your research.

Thesis – a thesis or position statement will show your planned message and should be worded so it can be included in the introduction and can be referred back to as a point to link the research and information to. If you were writing about body temperature reduction in surgical cases you would mention the importance of maintaining body temperature and the areas of nursing intervention where a difference can be made.

Tutor/supervisor – you will be assigned a member of staff with experience and expertise in the subject area to support you. They WILL NOT write this for you, but they are a sounding board for ideas and can direct you towards areas of recent work. If you are carrying out research related to vet nursing but it is non-clinical you may have a supervisor with knowledge in that area who isn't a vet or a nurse. This can be beneficial as they may see areas for research you had not considered but you may also need to spend time explaining the veterinary world to them so they can consider how your work could impact vet nurses.

Meaningful data

What do we mean by data? Data in this context is the information you have found by carrying out methodical research. You create numerical and contextual data (quantitative and qualitative) that needs to be reviewed through recognized frameworks to create solid evidence of the question you set out to answer.

What is relevant and meaningful data? You create relevant and meaningful data by creating a logical path from:

- the question you wish to answer
- your hypothesis
- your research strategy and methodology
- the way you analyse the data.

How can you find and collate data relevant to your subject area? By using:

- questionnaires
- studies
- recorded data from patients
- focus groups.

Please do not worry that at the start of your dissertation you may not know exactly how you will achieve all these stages. There are numerous books and websites to help you – check for some in the bibliography at the end of the book.

What will help you is to consider the stages that your work will go through. There is a helpful website (it requires a small subscription) at Laerd Dissertation

S T A R T	Stage 1	Stage 2	Stage 3	Stage 4	Stage 5	Stage 6	Stage 7	Stage 8	Stage 9	Stage10	E N D
	Getting to the main article	Choosing your route	Setting research questions / hypotheses	Assessment point	Building the theoretical case	Setting your research strategy	Assessment point	Data collection	Data analysis	Write up	

Figure 3.3 Laerd Dissertation

that takes you through each stage of your dissertation. It is very focused on your statistical side and links to a second website set up to help you navigate **statistics** and the software you will need to analyse the data you have. I find so many student vet nurses have a fear of maths and numbers – I cover working with numbers in Chapters Two and Five but for your dissertation make use of the tools available – there are a few and we'll look at them below.

From the timeline in Figure 3.3 you will see that the actual write up is listed as the final stage. While you cannot carry out a full write up until all the results are in I would suggest that you do start the writing process while you research your ideas. As with research for assignments the note making stage is often where you form your ideas and make new connections across the new information you find, so it is a good idea to not only make notes of potential quotes for supporting your theory but also to start recording your thought process and your ideas. Do not be afraid to start writing short paragraphs early on – these are especially handy if you can type them as they can then easily be edited and inserted into your main work.

This timeline also has two 'assessment points'. Do not worry – they do not mean that an external person comes and assesses your work at these points, but they are a good time for you to review where your journey is going and to meet with your supervisor to discuss this.

At assessment point one you will have set the question you wish to answer and have carried out your main reading. At this point you might find that your dissertation journey has already started to wander off the path you intended. Instead of battling on with your original idea and hoping it all works out, now is the time to decide where the journey is going – do you need to review the question you asked? Is there enough information to support the question you have set and do they use methodologies that you can use in your work? The research methodologies you read about should be the ones you aim to use, as this then puts your research in a similar category as the work that has gone before and you also know that ethics committees are more likely to approve the methodologies and that you will get valid results.

'Many of the truths that we cling to depend on our point of view.'
– Obi-Wan Kenobi, Star Wars VI
–The Return of the Jedi

The second assessment point is before you start your data collection, when you have finished your theory research and have decided on your research methods. At this stage, your research should have also been approved by the ethics committee and you will know where and when your research will be carried out and when it will have been completed.

Assessment at this stage should be to ensure you have created a research path that will provide valid results, and that you have all the appropriate approvals, that the other people involved know what they are doing and when. You have a theoretical case for the question and have noted the changes you made at assessment one. Yes, note the changes! Part of the learning process from original research is noting what you have changed through the process and why. This is why the assessment points, and you can add more in if you want to, are so important. It is normal to have to change things during the process of research, or to find out things you were not expecting to or to have data that does not fully support what you originally set out to do. Rather than ignoring these and hoping all will be well in the end – make life easier on yourself and make your final write up easier by acknowledging changes as you go along and noting why they happened and what you would do in the future to avoid them. This shows critical thinking and that you are reflecting on your work, both of which are very important, and one of the key things an assessor will be looking for.

Statistics – what help is there for you?

If you are worried about using statistics and how to analyse them please read this section. There are a number of software options to help and I have looked at a few of the most popular ones, SPSS, SAS, R and Python.

SPSS looks at first like a spreadsheet, but it is so much more. While you can enter data rather like using MS Excel you can include non-numerical data and the spreadsheet has multiple windows that allow you to view the data in a variety of ways, including looking at metadata.

While much software like this is very expensive, IBM, the developer, allows students free access for a short period of time or your college or university may pay for access. It is important to find out which access you may have. If you have a limited free access window you will need to be focused and make plenty of time to learn how to use it, input your data and get information from it you can work with. Although before you start work on the actual software there are excellent YouTube videos to prepare you.

It is worth checking some of these out before you design a questionnaire as they will let you see what SPSS will do with your data and, particularly for qualitative data, you may wish to review the options you give as answers to questions as SPSS is quite advanced in its analysis of qualitative data.

There are other software options and your college will be able to advise you if they have a preferred way of analysing data and if they have a subscription to let you use it for free or at a reduced cost. Remember to find out about these options early on in your project, as making sure you access all the help available at the best point in your journey requires forward planning.

Of the other software options the most popular are SAS, R and Python. Both R and Python are open access for the standard package so are free to use unless you need more advanced add on software. They all have their good and bad points and some are more suited to social science work and some to clinical work so do take some time to check out the options available to you as part of your research and reading at the start of your dissertation work.

> '*You will find only what you bring in.*'
> – *Yoda*, Star Wars: Episode V – The Empire Strikes Back

Literature reviews

You may have the choice of carrying out a literature review for your dissertation and I think many people feel this is the easier option – no ethics committees or data analysis, just a pile of journals and you passing your judgement on them. Get the kettle on, I'm writing my dissertation! Literature reviews for vet nursing do throw up their own problems and are not necessarily any easier than original research, it is a case of having a different set of problems to solve.

Even if you are carrying out an original research project, the following advice is useful. You will need to do a mini-literature review as part of your reading for your original research to demonstrate that there is a need for your research and also possibly identify more research that is required once yours has been completed.

A literature review is still a structured piece of writing and you still need to have a focus and a planned question to answer or specific area to review. I like these questions from the University of Toronto, they help to shape your main research question.

- What is the specific thesis, problem, or research question that my literature review helps to define?
- What type of literature review am I conducting? Am I looking at issues of theory, methodology, policy, quantitative research or qualitative research?
- What is the scope of my literature review? What types of publications am I using (for example, journals, books, government documents, popular media)?
- What discipline(s) am I working in (for example, nursing, psychology, sociology, medicine)? (University of Toronto, n.d.)

Using these four questions as a guide you can start to make decisions about how your review will work. Recently the volume of vet nursing-based academic work published has risen and so you would be able to look at some areas that would not have been possible before. Could you now review the effect of recent policy changes on veterinary nursing, or narrow the field by using only vet nursing/vet tech publications? For those who wrote their dissertation 5–10 years ago these options would not have been available.

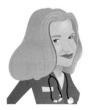

It's hard work but it's an exciting time to be carrying out original vet nurse research.

Reflective practice

Review and apply

Whether you realize it or not, **reflection** is an important part of writing. You need to review the research you have read to apply it to the question you are trying to answer. 'Reflection' is to be a word a lot of people do not warm to, and so suggest 'review and apply' is a more accurate and practical way to describe the process.

You need to review and apply the information you have found to your situation. You can do this by writing down ideas, creating mind maps, discussing ideas with colleagues, in fact in any way you want. You may want to check the downloadable reflective templates we have online.

Some practical ideas to help you, include heading back to Chapter One and looking at the different options there. There are some basic questions you can ask of your written work. This might seem odd but it can help you identify what you want to say.

Consider:

- who you are writing for
- what do you want to say
- why do you want to say that
- where, when and how did you get the evidence to support your ideas on what you are saying.

This will make you start to reflect or review your written work. It will help you to formulate ideas and opinions and start to help you read your work as a tutor may read it. While what we write makes sense to us as we know the full story, it can sometimes be hard to get across to the reader all that we want to say – coherently and in the required style.

Taking time to review your work is essential. Remember the sandwich anatomy from earlier in this chapter. Reviewing, editing and re-writing can take as long as the initial writing, if not longer. Figure 3.4 repeats the reflective cycle from Chapter One but has been adapted to show you that it can be applied to your research as well as practical experiences at work. It is part of the process of writing and starts your editing process.

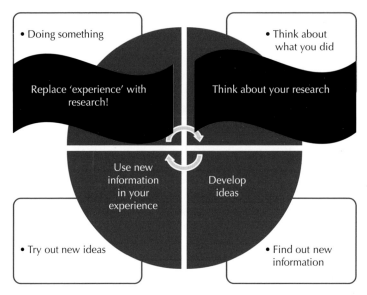

Figure 3.4 Kolb's Learning cycle (1984) in Solent (2017) – adapted for assignment writing

Editing your work

Editing is a really useful and important thing to do and is as important as writing. Knowing that you will later return to edit your work frees you to write. You can address links between each part when you are editing. Later, when you are required to produce longer pieces of work it is unlikely you will be able to produce a well written, balanced piece of work by writing straight through from introduction to conclusion. You will need to write, review and edit as you write, and once you have completed your writing and have put everything in your preferred order.

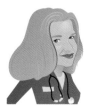

Start editing with simple tasks. Reading work aloud helps you hear if it makes sense.

Reading aloud is particularly useful if you are having difficulty phrasing some sentences. We are often clearer when speaking than when writing. If you have someone to read work to, even better. Unless they are an amazing friend or family member they are unlikely to want to sit through a 3,000-word assignment reading session. Try and focus on areas you really need help with to make the most of everyone's time.

Getting someone else to read your work is also helpful. They do not need to have knowledge of the subject area as they can still input on lay-out, spelling, grammar and punctuation. Even if they do not have knowledge of the subject area they will still also be able to recognize if you are using an academic style, appropriate language. Sometimes a reader not sharing your specialist knowledge is helpful, it they can understand it and the argument proposed makes sense to them then you are obviously making good progress.

As I have mentioned before please ensure you leave time for editing. Rushing this at the end can lead to lower marks as you have not presented your work as well as it could be. I definitely did not spend as long editing this book as I would have liked!

Harvard referencing and citation

Let us finish the chapter on a student favourite – even more fun than reflection – Harvard referencing.

What is it?

Any referencing system is a way of showing how your reading has influenced your thoughts and ideas on the subject. You need to give evidence of this and so referencing is a standardized way to show this evidence in your written text without interrupting the reading flow. You then link the citations to a full list of the materials used that gives all the information a reader needs.

Confusingly, both mentions of the text you read are called a 'citation' with the version in the text usually called 'short citation' and the one in your reference list called the 'full or long citation'. Alternatively, the mentions in the text may be referred to as the 'citation' and the full details as the 'reference' or bibliographic entry.

You do not have to memorize how to Harvard reference! Make sure you keep a copy of the examples and use them when you need to complete you referencing.

There are numerous referencing systems and your college or university will advise you which they use but it is likely to be based around the popular Harvard, or author–date, referencing system. They will be able to provide you with examples of system being used for books, websites and online journals. Common alternatives include foot or endnotes with or without short titles, or numbered reference indications, as superscripts or numbers in square brackets, both followed up with a reference list at the end.

Why do we use it?

While it is more work for you using a referencing system it is the only way to ensure that those reading (and marking) can see what you have read and how this has influenced you. It prevents you plagiarising the works you have read and provides an easy way for people to read around the subject area.

It is highly likely that your use of references will be on the marking criteria, particularly for undergraduate courses. This means your referencing can affect the grade you get. Using Harvard referencing is not a memory task, it is simply looking at a template for presenting information and applying it to your work. It takes time and attention to detail – and at the end of an assignment you may not have much of either.

The process starts with your research as you are likely to be graded on two aspects of Harvard referencing:

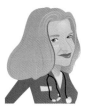

Do not let poor referencing drag your marks down – make time to reference.

- the quality of the research you have found – check out Chapters One and Two on digital literacy/critical thinking
- the presentation of your evidence, that is, are your full stops and commas in the right place and do you use citations correctly?

On the former, digital literacy does need some work and Chapter Two will help you start to critique the information you find. For the latter, citations and reference lists, keep reading here.

How do you do it?

This book uses Harvard referencing. As I have said above, do not think that you have to memorize how to Harvard reference. You only need to use it for course work and *not* in exams. You will always be able to consult your college or universities guide – but do leave time for this so you do not rush it and face losing marks with simple errors. Think back to the assignment sandwich (Figure 3.1) and check the time you have planned. The writing may take less time than you think and the research, editing and referencing will probably take longer.

Harvard referencing can feel confusing when you are writing – when should you put the authors name in for a short citation and should it be in brackets or as part of the text? You need to cite the source of any idea or statement that has come from your reading. The following list will give you some ideas:

- inspiration/thought process supporting
- theory supporting
- supporting statistics and data
- direct quotes
- paraphrasing.

There are many good guides to Harvard referencing on the web, for example, this one from Great Ormond Street Hospital (https://www.ucl.ac.uk/child-health/support-services/library/library-support-students/guide-harvard-citation-style), which covers the main type of in text citation and goes on to give examples of full reference for the different types of publication referenced. It is important to note that Harvard referencing is the underlying mechanism, the style of how the information is presented will vary from publication/institution to publication/institution. You will need to check any guidelines available. For example, (Bloggs, 2000: 102) or (Bloggs, 2000, p 102) or whether book/journal titles are in italics or plain (roman) typeface in the bibliography.

While you make notes, it is worth ensuring you keep the notes from one source clearly marked and separate from other notes. Where you find themes or contradicting information, keep another document of ideas about the subject to see what you are learning. In this document, it is worth making sure that you write the papers where you got the information so you end up with a main 'ideas' document that then leads you to the information you have pulled from that document. This sounds like a lot, but it really helps you as ideas do not get confused and you do not get set on an argument to build in an assignment then cannot find the great quotes that back it up.

Your citations are then easier to write, as you have them in note form already. As I said in Chapter Two keep a list of what you have read, including the dates accessed and the URL if an online text.

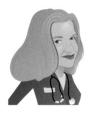

Copy & Paste is going to be your friend for creating reference lists!

To give you an idea of how I have been working with references for this book – the box contains my working reference list for Chapter One.

Example of a reference list in progress

RCVS 2015 Code of Conduct. Web page accessed 5.12.16
http://www.rcvs.org.uk/advice-and-guidance/code-of-professional-conduct-for-veterinary-nurses/supporting-guidance/delefation-to-veterinary-nurses/

Rowling, J.K., 1998. Harry Potter and the Chamber of Secrets. Bloomsbury: London

Rowling, J.K., 2000. Harry Potter and the Goblet of Fire. Bloomsbury: London

Jasper. M, 2003. Beginning reflective practice. Nelson Thornes Cheltenham

Teekman exploring reflective thinking in nursing practice 2000 j of adv nursing 31(5) 1125–1135

Cottrel, S., 2013. The Study Skills Handbook. 4th Ed. Palgrave McMillan: Hampshire

http://learn.solent.ac.uk/mod/book/view.php?id=2732&chapterid=1112

Kolbs Learning cycle (1984) in Solent (2017)

Pelzer and Hodgson, Vet Med Ed 2017 p 66

It includes books, webpages, online journals, print journals and a website. None of these are yet in perfect Harvard referencing style, but the information is all there so when it comes time to submit my work I can get out the agreed referencing style and add the full stops, tweak the commas and make things italic if they need it. This will still take time, but I do not need to start researching again to find the work I used, so the extra time taken during my research and writing will really help me here.

As you get familiar with your referencing system you will get better – I can always recall the correct way to space out Surnames. Initials., And Year but after that I always need to check – which is absolutely fine. The tutor does not see this work in progress they see the final version so however you manage it, just make sure you do tidy it up.

There are online reference generators to help you. While these can be seen as a great way to save time, the free ones still require you to know what information is needed and you have to input it. They do not really save you time and if you have relied on these at the end of your work you may find you are missing the country or publisher and have to spend time hunting for this.

An easier way to prevent you having missing information is to construct your own table to fill in with data as you research – Excel can offer a large template that is easy to use, or Google Docs is also helpful. Figure 3.5 is a rough example of using a Google Docs table to record your research.

Author	Author	Author	Year	Article title / Chapter	Journal / Book title	Online – webpage / pdf title Print – journal no / vol	URL	Date access	Country	Publisher
Davidson, J.	na	na	2017	Veterinary nursing uniforms: their role in infection control	The Veterinary Nurse	Jane Davidson The Veterinary Nurse, Vol. 8, Iss. 1, 24 Feb 2017, pp. 6010	http://www. theveterinary nurse.com/ cgi-bin/go. pl/library/ abstract. html?uid=10 8161	1.7.17	UK	Mag

Figure 3.5 Example of reference list

Before it makes you worry about the amount of information you need to collate to reference properly – I could copy and paste pretty much all the information here. This took less than a minute and has given me all the

> *'May the Force be with you.'*
> *– Yoda,* Star Wars: Episode IV –
> A New Hope

information I need to reference it in the style needed when the time comes. Copy and pasting this also means it's less likely to distract you from the thought process you are in about the information you have found. This way of working is that you focus on the information found and do a 'data dump' of the information you will need later. You could even copy this table to the top of your notes page for each item you read – meaning at the end you just need to copy and paste the top of each page used to a separate list to create your reference list.

It really is that simple to Harvard reference easily – you just need a little bit of planning and to make sure you leave enough time to complete it fully.

I hope from this chapter you can see the skills for academic writing are achievable. The skills differ from those used for exams and you can create the time and space to allow you to succeed. Now let us move on to look at exam skills.

 Review Chapter 3 and how to apply what you have learned with the Reflective Template.

Chapter Three glossary

academic writing – the presentation of your work in a formal writing style

citation – an indication that a resource has been used in the content of an assignment for example, 'Davidson (2017) states'

dissertation – extended writing assessment usually associated with an undergraduate degree course

ethics – ethical considerations are required for original research dissertations

feedback – verbal or written communication of an assessment of your work

grammar – the rules and guidelines covering the correct and preferred use of language, ensure clear communication

literature review – searching for and presenting the available current information

meaningful data – data that can be applied in the way you planned

paragraphs – a mini-essay on one part of the subject area

plagiarize – using someone else's work as your own

punctuation – , . ! ? : ; simplistically, the traffic lights that control writing

reflection – the process of considering your thoughts and actions to improve them in the future

sentences – a set of words that is complete in itself, the convey a single idea

statistics – numerical data

syntax – related to grammar, the arrangement of words and phrases to create well-formed sentences

third person – the expected style of presenting your findings – use 'he/she/they' instead of 'I/me/you'

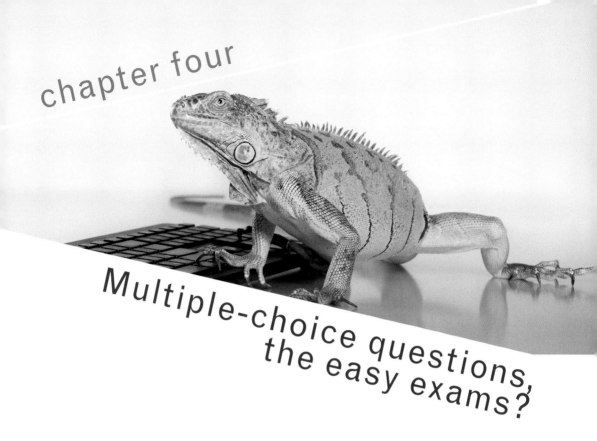

chapter four

Multiple-choice questions, the easy exams?

Multiple-choice question (MCQ) exams are the one many people dread, but is that a reflection of the exam style or the subject area it is most commonly used in? MCQ exams are commonly used for vet nurses, vets and in the medical field in general so you are not alone in sitting these exams. They are different to standard essay-style exams and require some time spent practising the style of exam as well as knowing the subject area.

MCQs are a successful exam style, for tutors, course designers and for students. I know this is hard to believe but statistically students will get higher scores in MCQ exams than in written assessments or long-answer exams.

This is because it is possible to score 100% in an MCQ exam but this is less likely in a written exam and almost impossible in an assignment. Therefore, it is considered a fair assessment, especially for larger subject areas where multiple assessment methods are used.

Subjects that are commonly assessed with MCQ exams include anatomy and physiology. This is a subject area people sometimes struggle with, so they associate MCQs with hard exams, when the subject matter is also difficult. It is worth spending time to find out which is the biggest hurdle for you – the subject or the exam style. I have found students admitting they have not pre-pared as well for an MCQ exam as they would for a written exam. This can be because they are not sure how to prepare for the exam style or because they think that with correct answers in there they do not have to do as much work before the exam.

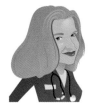

Think MCQs are the easy exams?
Do not fall for this fallacy!

The style of MCQs and how they are written is different to open-ended essay questions and you need to become familiar with the closed style of question-ing. This can feel difficult as we generally use open questions when talking, so to narrow things down feels very different.

The difference is that an open question wants the person answering to give a lot of information – questions are asked that allow someone to speak or write freely. While MCQs are not truly closed questions – that is, questions that only allow a Yes or No answer, they do focus on the information given in the answers.

It is worth bearing in mind that it is extremely rare to enter an exam and know 100% of all the aspects of the subject area. Yes, in an MCQ exam it is technically possible to get 100% and in short revision quizzes of 10–20 MCQs it is possible but in an exam with over 100 questions it's less likely. Another difference between MCQ and written exams, in written exams we do not see what we do not know as we focus on writing what we do know. You might need a slightly different approach and attitude to succeed with MCQs so that you do not get a nega-tive feeling when you do not know an answer instantly and start the negative spiral that makes you less confident in your answers which then reduces your confidence and can impact on your ability to do well in an exam.

'There'll come a moment when you think you can make it, and you'll try.'
– Robert Ludlum, The Bourne Identity

Head to Chapter Five and check out the Exam Prep Timetable I have adapted from Stella Cottrell to help you prepare for any exam, but now let us look in depth at MCQs.

What are MCQs?

MCQs are, as their name suggests, questions where you are given the answer. How amazing is that! If all the correct answers are there for you then why do people fail, and why do really 'clever people' not get 100%?

Well, because the questions and answers are set up to require a certain level of knowledge. Just because the correct answer is in front of you does not mean it is easy for you to spot, unless you have done the work and know the subject area. There are no easy questions, there are just answers you know, answers you can work out, and answers you do not know.

The questions can sometimes be simple in their wording but they can also contain supporting information to help you – and when reading quickly in the stress of an exam situation you might miss the important parts of the question. To make full use of the information provided then consider how you recall information for exams.

As noted earlier, Strauss et al. (2010) has noted three different levels of knowledge.

- Cognitive resonance – what we do know and can recall.
- Cognitive dissonance – what we know we should know but do not/cannot recall.
- The gaps where we did not know there was something to know.

Where MCQ exams help you is with cognitive dissonance, where we may struggle to recall something. If there is supporting information in the answers it can help you work out the answer, but only if you know your subject area. With this in mind, remember not to allow you nerves to affect you so much that when you see unfamiliar words or phrases it puts you off. You do know what you have revised and very few people go into an exam knowing 100% of the answers.

With the idea that MCQs can actually help you pass your exam, let us address some of the myths about this particular exam style.

When are MCQs used?

MCQs are used in many subject areas and for different reasons. As I have already mentioned they provide a very focused way of assessing information.

Responding to MCQs is a skill that you need to learn and so you may find you sit short MCQ tests as your module or course progresses. They are used both to help you get better at reading and answering MCQs and also so you can see how well you understand a small section of the information you have recently learned. Your tutor will also use the results to gauge how well you are doing with your studies. The tutor can also try out new questions and styles of questioning in these smaller tests before using them in a final exam.

MCQs can be used as final assessments in modules. Where you have been assessed by other means, written exams, assignments, practical exams, an MCQ exam is an opportunity to increase the overall marks gained for a module. It is true that students will score higher marks in MCQs than in most other assessments they sit. Therefore, it is important that you see them as an opportunity to do well.

When you are qualified and completing your CPD you will find MCQs often used as proof of learning. This can be at the end of articles in journals, or at the end of online modules. More recently, online CPD courses have started asking for MCQs to be completed to a certain pass mark. This then is evidence of learning and allows access to the all important CPD certificate.

How they help you

As the MCQ style of exam is very precise it can feel unforgiving. There are no marks for presenting wider information about the question asked, as happens in written exams. If you do not know the exact information asked for, you will struggle. You should, and in fact I urge you to *always*, put an answer even when you are unsure, as the chance of it being successful is then only dictated by the number of answers available – for four answer questions you have a 25% chance of getting it right. If you really do not know the answer it's better than a 0% chance of getting it right. However, you will not pass an exam by scoring 25%, so reserve this strategy for the questions that have you truly stumped.

We note why they are used above, but apart from getting you higher marks how else can they help you?

They are focused on one area. This helps you spend your time wisely when revising. Your revision is also less likely to need in depth reading and research. This does not mean you can scan information quickly, but that the style of questioning is usually based on facts and less on your opinions or views. Therefore, your time will be spent learning from resources you can find easily rather than trying to find out new information and ideas.

The style of the exam means it is not usually seeking your opinion or view on the subject area, the exam is set up to show your knowledge. For some people this is an exam style they prefer as they can stick to the facts and information that is black and white.

As you will be ticking a mark sheet or clicking a mouse to enter the information, MCQs are not an assessment or reflection of your writing skills. Some people feel they struggle with writing essays in exams and find MCQs or even the short-answer written exams less stressful.

> 'One balks, then agrees, then balks again only to agree again; that is the way one learns things.'
> – Robert Ludlum, The Bourne Identity

Different assessment styles are used across courses so there are styles to suit everyone. Even if MCQs are not your preferred style they are useful to help you gain higher marks – if you prepare well. Before we start looking at how we approach this style of exam let's get through some of the common myths there are about them.

MCQ myths busted

There are a number of myths surrounding MCQ exams, some people feel they are written to trip you up, or make the answers hard to work out. They really are not, but they do require that you know your subject very well. There is no opportunity to talk or write generally about the subject and show other knowledge to support your answer. You cannot gain extra marks from including information not directly related to the question. You either are right or wrong. It can feel very unforgiving, but let us look at a few of the commonly stated issues with MCQs.

Some questions are easier than others

While there can be different levels of assessments depending on your course or year of study, the questions presented are of the level required. There will be questions that are meant for the majority to answer, and some that only a few may know, but there are always enough of the former to allow everyone to pass if they have done enough work. Later I will discuss how to construct your own questions and answers so you can practice at home.

> *You either know the answer, and so the question is 'easy' or you do not know the answer so the question is 'hard'.*

Overlapping ranges

If ranges are given, for example, for temperatures, then the ranges offered as answers should not overlap. This causes confusion. If you think they overlap, then carefully re-read the answers and also the **units** given.

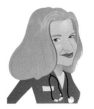

> *UNITS – yes meant to be in capitals – are a big stumbling block in many exams so do not forget to check them when you select your answer.*

Wording

The wording of the questions can seem a little unusual. They are direct, closed style questions and as such are very different from the way we usually communicate. Make sure you read the question carefully and that you understand the **stem**. The stem is the problem or question they wish you to answer. While other information may be given to create a scenario or to guide you, make sure you focus on the stem of the question. This is a good example of a question that offers information in the question that can help you – if you read it carefully.

Which of the following tumours affecting bone and associated tissues is benign?

A   osteosarcoma   C   osteochondroma

B   fibrosarcoma   D   chondrosarcoma

Here the simple stem is 'Do you know what an osteochondroma is?'. You are being given extra information, but do not let that distract you. It can be easy to scan read this question and fit it to what you know or what is most familiar, for example, to see the words 'tumour' and 'bone' and head straight to 'osteosarcoma' without reading what the question wants.

Even if you are not confident in this area the way the question is constructed gives you useful information – if you did not know what an osteochondroma was, but you knew sarcomas are not benign then you would get this right. More proof that you should not be put off when you see words you do not know in an exam.

There is more on this type of question later in this chapter.

Do you have enough time to properly read the question and review the answers?

Many people think you have a lot of spare time in an MCQ exam. This is because you get adequate time to:

• read
• answer
• review.

The exam provides enough time for you to read each question fully, choose the correct answer and review your answers. Many people finish MCQ exams in less time than is provided. This can be because they really knew their stuff, they had practised the question style and were very organized. Or it can also be because they rushed the reading and reviewing.

Everyone can use the exam time as they wish – you do not get any more marks for finishing fastest and there is little correlation between the time taken in an exam and the ability to pass it.

With the computer-based exams becoming more common, the reviewing of questions has become easier as you can go through the questions you wish to check much more quickly than with a paper-based exam. Use the practice session you get with online exams to help you move around the exam quickly and build confidence.

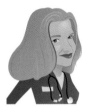

People who finish an exam quickly are not necessarily the most successful.

False answers

The 'false' answers or **distractors** are not made up names or there to trip you up. They are chosen as alternatives that include information or terminology from the same subject area, that are true statements, but are not the correct answer to the question. Unlike an essay question, you cannot simply state all that you know and link it to the question. You can use the four answers given to help you – as they give you other words/information from the same subject area. Use what you know about all the answers given, to narrow the options down to the correct one, and if there are two that are similar, read them carefully and check the wording, the numerical content and any units of measurement – yes UNITS again.

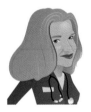

UNITS UNITS – CHECK THE UNITS – UNITS UNITS.

Changing answers

Yes – you will feel the need to change answers when reviewing your exam paper. Reading questions a second time can lead you to think your answer is incorrect. In all the years I have been teaching I have watched as countless people later realize they have changed a right answer to a wrong one. The frustration! However, you do not recall with as much horror when you have changed wrong to right – so is your memory playing tricks on you? Well, possibly.

A study in 1984 showed that almost 53% of students felt changing answers would lower the marks gained (Benjamin et al. 1984). From my experience, students do not always feel this is the case. If you read the question again and feel strongly that you have the wrong answer then change it. The rest of this chapter should help you to improve your skills so that you make the first choice the right choice.

Was it the questions or your revision that were the problem?

Often students come out of an exam and say 'it was all equine' or 'it was all endocrine'. They feel that the questions were weighted towards one particular area, and in each case it was an area they were not as prepared for as they could be. As with all exams, MCQ exams are monitored closely when they are created. There will be a bank of questions that have been moderated and checked. These are then chosen for exam papers. The number of subject areas within the overall exam subject area is monitored.

What actually happens is the questions you know and answer easily you forget. You read them once and then moved on. The questions you recall are the ones you had to read more than once, that is, the ones for which you did not know instantly and had to read again. Hence, they stick in your mind. You may still have the answer correct, you just are not as sure as for some of the other questions. These questions and subject areas stand out and worry you. This is perfectly natural. We all have areas we think we do not know as well as others, that we did not understand as easily as we would like – that is normal. It does not mean the exam was set up to make you fail, it did what exams do – showed up the areas you were weaker in. This does not mean you have failed. You should take the indications of your weaker areas forward to other assessments and prepare better.

'But I only failed on 3 questions'

When the results come out and students have failed by a tiny margin I've often heard the cry 'I only failed by 3 questions'. Yet few exams have a pass mark of 90–100%. For many MCQs the pass mark is 50% or 65%. If you did not pass then there are a lot of questions you failed on. If an exam has 100 questions and a 65% pass mark then you failed on more than 35 questions – that is more than one-third of the exam. While your brain will focus on the few questions you can recall that you were worried about it is not this small area that needs work, but a much larger review of all the subject matter. This is not meant to be harsh – failing an exam is hard, especially if you were close to passing. Aiming to achieve 'just a pass' is a poor strategy. All you need to do on the day is come across a few questions you are not sure of, some where you make a mistake typing in your answer, and some that you misread and put the wrong answer and you fail. The exam has shown your weaknesses, just as it was designed to do – use this information to help you.

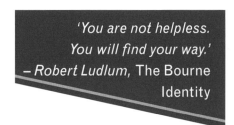

'You are not helpless. You will find your way.'
– *Robert Ludlum*, The Bourne Identity

How to answer an MCQ

Answering an MCQ starts with reading the question carefully, ensuring you understand what is being asked. When you have a lot of information to process in a stressful situation it can help to narrow down what you are seeing.

Covering the answers while you read the question may help to prevent you from scanning the question quickly while selecting the wrong answer. It slows down your reading speed and makes you focus on the question. There will be spare, blank paper in an exam to allow you to make notes or write down workings and you can use this to cover the part of the screen should you need to.

When reading the questions you will find some recurring question types:

Which of the following is true . . .
Which of the following is false . . .
Most correct . . .

For anatomy questions you may also find questions based on anatomical directions.

The anterior surface of the liver rests:

A   On the caudal surface of the diaphragm
B   On the caudal pole of the right kidney
C   In contact with the loop of the duodenum
D   Against the lesser curvature of the stomach

There may be extra information in the question. This is there to guide you and help narrow down the correct answer options. If you read the question and then the answers and feel there are two possible options, then the clue to working out which is correct will be in the wording of the question.

Which one of the following best describes an increase in white blood cells on microscopic examinations?

A   Leucopenia
B   Leucocytosis
C   Haemolysis
D   Hypochromic

(City and Guilds Sample Paper 2017
available to SVNS registered with C&G)

This question stem contains three points of information:

• increase
• white blood cells
• it is for a microscopic examination.

These are not there to confuse you but to give you enough information to choose the correct answer.
    If you do not know the answer you may be able to work it out by a process of elimination. The question narrows the field of information and to get to the correct answer you should take time to consider information related to the

specific question area. With the question above you could use your knowledge of:

- prefixes: haem-, leuco-, hypo-
- suffixes: -penia, -cytosis, -lysis
- names of diseases involving white blood cell levels
- knowledge of microscopy.

For the previous question on the position of the liver you could call on your anatomical knowledge of the:

- kidneys
- diaphragm
- duodenum
- stomach
- anatomical direction.

So, you now have a strategy to work out individual questions. What are you going to do for your overall approach to the exam? If you do not know the answer to a question what will you do? You already have the SQ3R process from Chapter Two to help you recall information (Boyd, 2014): Survey, question, read, recall, review.

This can be altered to RAIF for MCQ questions:

- Read
- Answer
- If not sure
- Flag and move on.

There are several reasons for moving onto the next question if you cannot answer the one you are on.

It is better to get into a flow in the exam and you will gather momentum, and build your confidence, by answering a number of questions successfully at the start of the exam. Just as in a written exam you would choose the exam questions you know best, you can do this in MCQ exams by flagging those you are unsure of and moving on.

You may also find that there is another question on the same or similar area later in the exam that helps you recall information in a way that helps answer a question you were previously stuck on. As your confidence grows you will feel more relaxed in the exam and you will be able to recall more; the difficult questions will begin to get easier.

This is also a good use of your time. While it is rare to run out of time in an MCQ exam it is a good exam technique to complete your strongest areas first when you are fresh and have the most energy. Better to run out of time on a question you were not sure of and may have got wrong, than on one you knew the answer for but rushed and got wrong or did not have time even to attempt.

By spending time wisely, answering all that you can answer and going back to the ones you cannot, you then leave time to work through the questions you could not answer easily on the first reading.

Reading the questions accurately

Anyone who has sat an MCQ test will tell you that there are three main issues:

- reading the question correctly
- reading the answers correctly
- whether to change answers when you review your answers.

Reading accurately is key to understanding what the questions ask of you. While some questions are straightforward:

Nephrectomy is the removal of:

A   a kidney
B   the oviducts
C   an adrenal gland
D   the deferent ducts
         (City and Guilds Sample Paper 2017 Available to SVNs with C&G)

Others give you more information that can help, and hinder you. The part of the question you are trying to answers is the 'stem' – the question subject area. There may be multiple questions on one stem area, for example, anatomy and physiology – orthopaedic issues/tumours. All with different answers. The stem may be clear, as in the example above. The question is set out with no extra information and is easy to understand.

Some questions contain more information. Look at the example below from earlier in the chapter:

Which of the following tumours affecting bone and associated tissues is benign?

A   osteosarcoma
B   fibrosarcoma
C   osteochondroma
D   chondrosarcoma

This question offers quite a lot of information. The stem is asking if you know what an osteochondroma is but is giving you information to help filter the answers. If you had not heard of osteochondroma, but knew your suffixes and prefixes well and knew that an osteosarcoma was malignant you could work out the answer.

This is sometimes why people come out of an MCQ exam and say there were questions on things they didn't know. There may be unfamiliar words and terminology and the way information is presented may not be what you are expecting.

As I have noted earlier in the chapter, with complex stem questions it can be easy to scan read them and not fully realze what the question is asking and then chose an incorrect answer. In contrast to questions with short, clear stems, which are quick to read, for questions with longer stems and more information you need to slow down and focus on the questions that give you further information. You are given enough time in this style of exam to give each question the attention it deserves.

Different styles of questions

There is the 'Which one is not' question, asking you to spot the odd one out from a list. This style of question is becoming less common as the wording has been deemed confusing for some. There should never be a double negative in the question or between question and answer. This type of question may also be phrased as 'which is X except'.

There is a commonly used phrase of 'Which is best/appropriate'. This is used in some areas of theatre or nursing care where we know there is more than one way of completing a task but also that there is a prescribed standard that has been researched and has evidence to support it. This can be seen in questions such as the following example.

What is considered an appropriate hand scrub time for the first scrub of the day using a standard antiseptic solution?

A   one minute
B   two minutes
C   three minutes
D   five minutes

In this subject area, we know that this information depends on several factors including the vet surgeons training, the products used for the first scrub and the products used after the first scrub. Therefore, the question is phrased to show this may not be the same in all practices but in an ideal situation where evidence based criteria are applied. You should also note in this question that some important information is given at the end of the question 'standard antiseptic solution'. While the start of the question states this question is about hand scrub you need two pieces of information to get to the answer:

• confirmation this is a sterile scrub technique rather than hand hygiene
• what product is used.

Do not fall into the trap of seeing the question is about sterile scrub technique and think 'in my practice we use X product and the time is X minutes' because you may use a different product and the scrub time may be different. Clearly, using brand names

> '*The easiest thing in the world is to convince yourself that you're right. As one grows old, it is easier still.*'
> – *Robert Ludlum*, The Bourne Identity

in a professional exam is not appropriate so do know your antiseptic and dis-infectant generic types as well as the brands.

Choices – the correct answers

In MCQ terminology the correct answer is known as the **choice**. The one you should choose. When writing MCQ exams, correct answers should be presented that are all the same length, so if the answer is one word or a short phrase all the distractors are written to mimic this. The myth that correct answers are 'always C' is sadly wrong as correct answers are spread evenly across all options – for four-answer exam styles and those with more answer options.

Distractors – the incorrect answers

These should always be written using real terminology and information. It must be true information that could be a correct answer in different circum-stances. They are not there to cause confusion but to allow you to demonstrate the depth of your knowledge. The following question is an example of using distractors to test your knowledge of several different areas.

Which of the following statement on muscle tissue is true?

A   Smooth muscle is striated
B   Skeletal muscle is voluntary
C   Cardiac muscle is non-striated
D   Smooth muscle is in-voluntary

(Muralitharan and Peate, 2001; this a book on human anatomy so not all questions will be accurate for veterinary work – answer is D)

It is offering information on:

- smooth muscle
- skeletal muscle

- cardiac muscle
- construction of muscles
- movement of muscles.

To be confident answering this question you would need to know the correct answer and be confident that the three other answers were incorrect. That means having a knowledge of all types of muscle.

Distractors need to be from the same subject area, not just drawn from random information. The question above is a good example of using information from the subject area to examine knowledge of several aspects of muscles.

The distractors can be drawn from common errors made by students. However much we like to think our journey as a student is individual to us there are areas where students commonly make mistakes. This can be with terminology that is spelt similarly – for example, epistaxis/epistasis, or areas where 'myths' are seen as the truth – especially in nursing care.

MCQs are useful in allowing large areas of the syllabus to be focused on while giving it the equal weighting of an MCQ. MCQs should provide at least three alternatives to the choice answer. Some courses have MCQs that provide six answers and this allows for a wider spread of knowledge to be assessed.

If the correct answer is not immediately obvious MCQs allow for a process of elimination. If you can't see the right answer straight away don't panic, and work through what each of the answers mean independently of the question being asked. This will stop you getting confused and is a positive thing to do as it will make you feel more confident as you know what the answers mean. Then go back and re-read the question and see if you can spot the right answer.

Calculations in MCQs

MCQ exams may contain calculations and while you will still select an answer from the four options given you will need to do the actual calculation. You

Nothing harms your confidence like entering an exam room and knowing that you have not prepared properly.

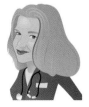

will be provided with a calculator and pen and paper in the exam. Yes, you can 'guess' but why take the risk? Plan to enter the exam being able to attempt every question.

Again, I would advise writing down any calculations you think you need once the exam starts. Use the spare paper provided and note the calculation. Once you have done this you do not need to worry about remembering it and it will also stop you trying to do part of the calculation in your head when you reach that question.

Then make sure you write down the *units* used. Although your answers will have units are they the correct ones?

We know in other exams that showing your working is as important as writing down the correct answer, yet in MCQs you can guess and avoid the maths, right?

Wrong! The distractors in the MCQ answers may have some obvious errors that you will only spot if you have done the maths. There can be differences between answers that are as simple as a moved decimal point or incorrect units. Yet these will not be obvious unless you have worked through the data given. See the example and working in the box.

Example

A young Chihuahua weighs 2 kg and requires a drug at a dose of 4 mg/kg/day split into two doses (BID).

The tablet strength is 8 mg. How many tablets are required per dose?

A   4 mg
B   8 mg
C   0.5 mg tablet
D   0.5 of a tablet

(Example from Moore and Palmer, 2001)

There are distractors here that are easy to pounce on. The question has a lot of information in it and it can be easy to scan read, see that the maths is quite simple and not read the end of the question and see what they are actually asking for. Not all drug calculations will require a final answer in mg/kg.

Working

2 kg × 4 mg/kg = 8 mg per day
dose is twice a day = 4 mg per dose
dose divided by tablet strength = 0.5 tablet

While this is an extreme example, the correct answer is D, it shows that you can have distractors that are the answer to some parts of the question that can easily mislead you.

It may help you in questions like these to take out the number data and make a note of it separately from the question:

Weight	2 kg
Dose	4 mg/kg/day
Tablet strength	8 mg

This means you can quickly check the data in your calculations is correct without getting stuck reading the whole question again. It keeps the numbers and words separate and this can be a big help if reading the question slows you down.

It also shows that the actual 'maths' part of the exam is often very simple and you might be able to do it without writing it down. While that is great, you do not get any more marks for that skill and may make an easy mistake through nerves and 'exam brain'. Therefore, I would strongly suggest you write down the working for each calculation in an exam, and check back through it – make sure you have the correct answer.

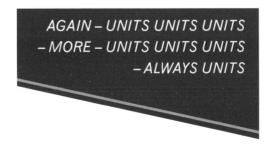

AGAIN – UNITS UNITS UNITS
– MORE – UNITS UNITS UNITS
– ALWAYS UNITS

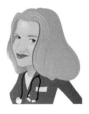

Extended MCQs and other MCQ options

After qualification, you will still face MCQs as they feature in CPD. They may include different MCQ options such as extended MCQs. Extended MCQs can take some different forms but they usually offer a more in-depth opportunity to assess knowledge. You may be given one or more stems carrying more information than a usual MCQ and be given five to seven options for the answer.

Revising and practising is the same as for pre-qualification MCQs, so you can use the skills from this chapter. You may need to practise reading questions carefully as the stems usually have more information and you have more answers to review. However, you do get allocated more time per question and they are used in addition to other assessment types, not entirely on their own.

Writing your own MCQs to aid revision

Making up your own MCQs to test yourself while you revise is a great idea. It helps reinforce knowledge and gets you thinking about the set-up of questions. Writing multiple MCQs can take some time. There are other similar question styles that can help you that are a little quicker.

I have used simple questions about terminology I could not recall easily. 'I used to find remembering the differences between gluconeogenesis and glycogenesis difficult'. I started with 'Which is glucose from a carbohydrate source?' as a question and progressed from there, adding layers of knowledge with each revision session.

This could then be developed into an MCQ as the information I gathered about the subject area could provide stems and distractors. With a simple search of similar terms, I found five related words that I researched and found the definitions for and linked them to the process of both the terms I was struggling with. I now have five distractors without trying too hard, and have learnt a little more in the process:

- glucokinase
- hexokinase
- glycolysis
- glycogenolysis
- glycogen.

You can then play around with using the appropriate terms in stems for questions.

Revising for MCQs – learning and memory techniques

How to prepare for an MCQ

Any exam requires you to know your subject area and therefore you must revise. The only difference with MCQs is that you are focusing less on your opinion on the information you have and more on the information itself. This means you need to be clear about what you know and understand. While some answers can help you use a process of elimination, sometimes they can confuse you so do not assume you need to do less work 'because you are given the answers'. While it is rare to get less than 40% in a written exam it is perfectly possible in an MCQ exam, and it is even possible to get 0%.

Revising for MCQs needs to focus on facts and how you can recall, compare and contrast them. Consider how a question could be posed to ask you the information you have just learned. You might start to spot potential distractors when there is similar information on the same subject area.

Make things as easy as possible and divide larger, complex areas into smaller, easier to recall areas. Memory aides might start to help here. Everyone is different but songs, rhymes and **mnemonics** can all help you recall information.

As mentioned elsewhere, you may also find it helps to make up your own MCQs to test yourself, and to see what an exam writer can see in the information you both have. You know already there is a stem, and a choice and three distractors, researching appropriate distractors is another way to find out new ways to remember information.

For example, I used to find remembering the differences between gluco-neogenesis and glycogenesis difficult. I used simple quiz questions initially, focusing on the difference that the first is related to glucose from a non-carbohydrate source and the second is storing glucose produce from a carb source. I started with 'which is glucose from a carbohydrate source?' as a question and progressed from there, adding layers of knowledge with each revision session.

The phrase 'Devil is in the detail' can be accurately used for MCQ exams. While you may know general information, or can remember details when

'I fought . . . I fought and I fought . . . until I . . . couldn't remember any more.'
– Robert Ludlum, The Matlock Paper

discussing cases, MCQs require you to know the subject area well and not to rely on the answers being in front of you.

This can feel quite daunting. Exams are not just memory tasks but you will need to feel comfortable working out the best way for you to recall information in a way that helps you in an exam.

Memory techniques

While you are learning facts for recall they can seem disconnected from what you do every day with your patients. To help you learn you can consider a few different approaches. Some of these can really help boost your study morale and make the whole experience seem more positive.

I like to use mnemonics. These are where you have a list of information and you take the first letter of each word and make an easy to remember phrase from it.

Objective structured clinical exams (OSCEs) can contain information you need to tell the examiner (see Chapter Seven). This can be hard to recall on top of actually doing the task. In imaging, you need to be able to demonstrate and tell the examiner your centring and collimation points. For the cervical spine this is:

- Cr – Occipital crest
- Ca – line of the 1st rib
- dorsal – skin surface
- ventral – about midline of neck
- centring on mid neck region.

This is a lot of information. When you have eight potential views to remember for this you need to be organized. List and remember the information so it always runs cranial, caudal, dorsal, ventral. This gives order to the information. Then take the actual points:

- occipital crest
- first rib
- skin
- about midline of neck.

Then take the first letter of each:

- O
- F
- S
- A.

Then make a phrase that is easy to remember: OSCE fear soon abates.
    Figure 4.1 provides another good example of creating a mnemonic.

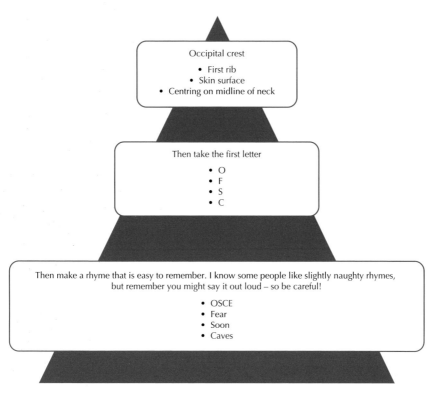

Occipital crest
- First rib
- Skin surface
- Centring on midline of neck

Then take the first letter
- O
- F
- S
- C

Then make a rhyme that is easy to remember. I know some people like slightly naughty rhymes, but remember you might say it out loud – so be careful!
- OSCE
- Fear
- Soon
- Caves

Figure 4.1 Mnemonics creator – an example

Notes

As for written exams where I advise writing down your own notes when the exam starts, notes of things you do not want to forget – I would advise the same for an MCQ.

This can help with your process of elimination as you have written down what you remember before being distracted by distractors. Once you have read a question it can be easy to make links to some or all of the answers and get confused. I have got some tips on avoiding that later.

> 'Opportunities will present themselves. Recognize them, act on them.'
> – Robert Ludlum, The Bourne Supremacy

My advice for making your own notes in the exam is to make them *before* you find the question on that area, ideally at the start of the exam. You know the subject areas the exam will cover, and can make an educated guess at what calculations you will need in advance, for example, for anaesthesia there are three common calculations. The information given in the question can help, but can hinder the memory process so make sure you are clear about what you are trying to recall. This is particularly true with calculations and numerical data. As the first step or two of many calculations can be done with mental arithmetic you easily start a calculation without writing it down and then get muddled about which step you have or have not done, so it is better to write out all the steps of any calculation you are working on as you go. This will also help you to spot any silly errors in your working.

Use the pen and paper provided in the exam and create a small box to put your notes in, to separate them from any workings or notes made during the exam. Or if you are provided with more than one sheet of note paper, use one for your notes and one for your working.

Songs and rhymes

The human brain works in many amazing ways. However, using our memory properly can be a challenge. We recall songs from the radio we have heard once but do not recall the functional parts of the kidney that we have spent hours reading about? There are many theories – including evidence that our brain processes music, lyrics and written words in a different way. Could making a rhyme or song about it help?

Songs can also help break down tasks into steps you can recall. The WHO hand wash has set steps that need to be completed in a set time. Can you get a short song or rhyme to fit?

For the six-step WHO hand wash you can use another song many people know – 'Jingle Bells':

1 Jingle palms, Jingle palms
2 Let's do back of hands
3 Interlace those fingers
4 and clasp to clean inside
5 thumbs next, left and right
6 then do finger tips
Then let those Jingle Palms dry

Other styles of rhyme that work well include rap songs or any familiar songs to you. You do not need to use the same songs as everyone else – use what works for you. Although bear in mind you will probably never recall the song the same again, so choose wisely. I do not want to be the reason you cannot listen to Beyoncé ever again.

Let us consider some of the reasons we can recall information presented via song or rhyme.

- There is muscle memory attached to singing along to music. Our brain is more likely to recall something where there are more triggers, such as a memory of reading, hearing and singing the same information. More of our memory works to recall this than information we have just read in silence.
- There is a location to recall when we heard the song. This triggers visual as well as auditory memory, again eliciting more of our memory stores to work.
- We listen to songs on more than one occasion so there is a repetition aspect that we need to use when revising and also we need to practise our recall once we have revised the information.
- We are more likely to recall information we have learned when we are relaxed or enjoying ourselves. Making your revision as stress free as possible will help. Finding a quiet, comfortable place to revise. Making sure you have eaten well, slept well.
- Putting your personality into your revision. Using colour, songs, pictures that all cheer you and create a positive atmosphere are all going to help you recall information – remember the CREAM acronym from Cottrell (2013) in Chapter One?

This is a good way to recall facts and figures. It can be hard to recall dates of legislation or other numerical facts. There is a well known children's rhyme that

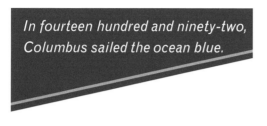

In fourteen hundred and ninety-two, Columbus sailed the ocean blue.

allows people to easily remember the year Columbus 'discovered' America which you can use as inspiration for making up your own memory aides.

It is simple, and easy. Do not be afraid to go back to basics with memory aides. They are for you and your learning needs, they do not need to be great works of poetry and you do not need to share them with anyone else if you do not want to.

Some examples of rhymes for numbers:

Veterinary Surgeons Act 1966
Since 66 they gave you meds for ticks.

COSHH 2002
Neutralising poo since 02.

Manual Handling 1992
Lifting safely for you, since 92.

Visual prompts

Everyone's style of learning is different. You may have already been identified as a visual learner. You may find it easier to recall information from coloured writing or images, and tables and diagrams may be easier to remember than lines of black writing.

Even if you already have printed notes or written notes you can change them into a more colourful version and can create more visually interesting revision. As with learning rhymes for facts, having colour themes for information can aid recall. Colours for subject areas, the importance of information and other ways of indicating extra information you need without having to write it down can all help.

You can introduce colour in many different ways. With pens for highlighting text, coloured writing for your own notes. Sticky notes that can be removed from library books, coloured paper or overlays to give textbooks or printed notes a different colour are also helpful. Those with dyslexia may be able to seek an assessment and find out which colour of printing and paper work best for you. For those that are not dyslexic you may still find moving away from black ink on white paper beneficial. The level of contrast between black ink and white paper is very high and reducing this contrast can make words appear more clearly. Even although I am not dyslexic I find navy ink on pale lilac paper a very calming combination that makes you want to read more.

Many colleges now print everything on cream paper and some only use blue ink for these reasons. If you think you have a learning need that could be helped with different coloured paper, overlays or ink then do speak to the learning support team at your college or university. As I mentioned in Chapter One it is your own journey and if you access help or support it is not gaining an unfair advantage, you are just sensibly getting the help you need. Take each chance to improve your achievement.

As I have mentioned, learning in a relaxed environment may help your recall. With visual learning, using positive, pleasant, nice images will increase your learning ability by encouraging that relaxed, engaging and possibly fun environment. I understand that especially for some programmes you may need to look at pictures of infected wounds and fractured legs: they are not fun or relaxing! However, they are part of your field.

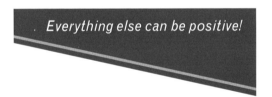

Everything else can be positive!

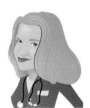

If you wish to use images in your learning, as it's for private use you may use some pictures that you find in books, or articles or the internet. Do remember that then you cannot share or post your revision notes anywhere if you have used copyrighted images. If you wish to share your notes then you can take your own pictures – with the required consent from the practice and owners. You can draw your own images for revision too. Line drawings and stick figures of animals will all work well and you can make up what you need. When making your own notes you also use more parts of your brain and also creative muscle memory and so increase your chances of recalling the information in the future.

As with rhymes or mnemonics anything that you find funny or a little naughty is likely to be remembered well. Though I suggest avoiding something you would be embarrassed for anyone else to read or overhear.

I have purposefully kept this 'visual section' free of images and you may wish to reflect on how well this section works for you as a learning tool of just text with few breaks.

One final visual option I use is criss-crossing words to help identify their meaning (Figure 4.2). Many of the words we learn in the veterinary field can be very similar, often as they are made up of a mix of prefixes and suffixes with only a few letters in the middle that make them different. This can be very hard to work with.

I'll use epistaxis and epistasis as my examples – similar spellings but with very different meanings. Presenting them side by side as they may be in an index or dictionary can be more confusing so write them down apart and consider the difference.

In this way, I can target the different spelling and put down a guide to the definition. Epistaxis is bleeding from the nose – expelling blood – and epistasis is the suppression of the action of a gene.

```
                E                          G                    P R A C T I C E
    E P I S T A X I S                      E                          O
                P                          N                          N
                E                          E                          C
                L                  E P I S T A S I S                   R
                L                          U                          E
                E                          P                          T
                D                          P                          E
                B                          R
                L                          E                    P R A C T I S E
                O                          S                          K
                O                          S                          I
                D                          E                          L
                                           D                          L
```

Figure 4.2 Crossword memory technique

Mind palaces

I first came to know about **mind palaces** through the character of Hannibal Lecter. While your mind is active with learning I will not advise stimulating it further by reading about a serial killer, but his use of mind palaces is worth considering. I will note that this form of recall and storing of information was new to me and it has been around since the early Greeks started using it in c.556–c.468 BC (Thomas, 2014). The theory is also known as the method of loci. Using locations of things or people to recall information. While you use this as locational learning in recalling where you first heard a song, or saw a band play, you can go a step further, using what you are learning to create a visual space in your mind. That you can move around and between items you choose to store there.

This might sound a little far-fetched but your mind has already started the process for you. When you try to recall information about what parasites praziquantel works on, your brain may visually take you to a time when you handled the packet, or read the instructions, or talked to someone about it. Instead of then getting side tracked with other memories from that time you can take what you recall and store it in your mind palace. In fact, you might want to put information for exams and work into a mind 'hospital'. Allowing you to walk around the spaces in your mind and store information in lab, theatre, dispensary and any other places that relate to the subject area. If you then need to recall information on a cat with renal failure, you can head to pharmacy for the medication, to the ward to check on fluid rates, the kitchen for nutrition. It is an alternative way to control how and where you file information in your brain. Again, it is personal to you and can be set up however you prefer, using cases you have seen and information you have learnt.

Aural memory

Using sound to promote memory and learning is a useful tool. As I have mentioned previously it seems odd that we can recall a song so easily after hearing it once on the radio but struggle to recall important facts we need to know. Could you create songs and rhymes as I have done above to help you remember?

While watching a video may seem like a visual aid, the audio that goes along with it may be easier to recall. Our brain stores audio and visual content separately and while they often are recalled together the sound of someone's voice may by more beneficial. Listening to people talking about a subject you are learning means you are getting the information you need but also hearing the tone and pace of the speakers and their emphasis on certain words can make remembering what is said much easier than just reading or watching videos with no audio.

This might not sound very library friendly but it is worth investing in a decent pair of headphones that are comfortable and will not disturb your neighbours while studying. Yes, we all have those free headphones from our mobile phones but they are not that great for comfort or sound quality, so although I do not advocate buying things you do not need and I am aware that finances are tight when you are a student, maybe ask for them as a gift for a birthday or Christmas. Using audio learning might just help you improve your grades.

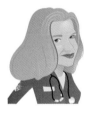

Podcasts and videos are still revision – if the content is relevant!

Practical experience

There is a lot of evidence that using real cases and learning information from a patient's journey is a great way to learn. As a student vet nurse you are guided to do this with your NPL/CSL. It has been shown that completing a log of cases seen improves success in achieving the course, especially with practical exams.

Pick some cases that are common, such as a new diabetic or thyroid case. Try to avoid the 'exciting' cases to focus on and go for ones that follow the normal patient journey from admission to diagnosis to treatment. These can then be used as a basis to find out more about the disease, the treatment and the progression over time.

It also means you are more informed about the patient and can answer owners' questions with confidence as well as increasing the level of nursing you can give that patient.

It is much easier and nicer to recall a patient you know and have a story about than just some figures in a text book.

You may wish to go over chosen cases with your clinical coach to ensure you are using the information the practice uses and match this with textbook theory.

Make up a story

The recurring theme of using stories to recall information is summed up here. You do not always need a song or a rhyme to put information in. A simple story could do to help remember facts.

I remember being told this as a memory technique in my student days. When learning what the parts of the X-ray tube head were and what they did we were told about Cathy cathode and Annie anode.

Cathy and Annie were out in a nightclub.

Where Cathy was running around causing a lot of negativity and making people move out of her way, Annie was being positive and helping usher people away from Cathy and towards the exit with its rotating door.

From reading this can you identify which part of the tube head is negative and which positive? You can add to and embellish these stories as much as you need to. I have included here information on the rotating 'door' for the anode. But you also have the focusing cup, target, focal spot, and other parts to learn.

This starts to help you recall where the anode and cathode are and what parts they play in producing X-rays. The technique is also helpful for anatomy and disease processes and can be linked to real cases.

Although focused on MCQs this chapter has also covered a lot of memory and recall techniques. These can be used for any exam style but are particularly useful for the precise nature of MCQs. I hope that this chapter lets you see that MCQs are not the exam style to be hated and feared – they can be conquered just like any other assessment style.

     More examples of memory aides are available online.

Other styles of short-answer exams

There are other styles of short-answer exams that you may see used.

True/false

These can be a good starting point in attempting to write MCQs. The stem is a simple statement and then the answers are 'true' or 'false'. There is then a 50% chance of being correct so if you test yourself using these make the 'pass' mark high.

While writing your true/false questions it will start to make you think of alternative answers and terminology that could be added to the correct answer.

Creating more answers that are false can be helpful as human nature will make us go for 'true' if we are not sure. Unlike MCQs it is best to avoid using negative statements and using words such as 'not'.

Matching

Matching questions put three to four options together and one is to be matched to the stem. This can be done with the same number of questions and answers – so there is a process of elimination or it can be done so that there are distractors.

Either way they are a simple way to set a test and something you may like to use as revision, even if you don't face them as an assessment.

On the day

When the day arrives, you will still feel nervous, no matter how much you have prepared. This is a good thing as you can use this nervous energy. Before the day make sure you know the basics.

- Where is the exam?
- Do you need identification to enter the exam?
- What do you wear?
- What do you need to do with hair or nails?

Check the exam prep checklist in Chapter Five. Have these things organized before the day.

Head back to Chapter One to see the advice on exam nerves and remember I find myself drawn again to the information from Straus et al. (2010) about knowledge gaps. I do not think anyone ever goes into an exam knowing 100% of all the information that can be asked. No matter how well prepared you are be aware that you will probably see questions or information that you do not recognize.

That is normal!

Do not let your confidence be knocked by one word in a question that does not immediately fall into place. That is not going to fail you an exam if you are well prepared.

Have your own mantra that you can repeat to focus on and ignore what else may be happening around you. You can make up your own but I like to remind students that the best thing to do is to breathe.

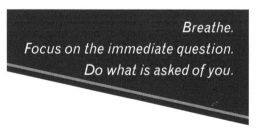

Breathe.
Focus on the immediate question.
Do what is asked of you.

Just breathe.

 Review Chapter 4 and how to apply what you have learned with the Reflective Template.

Chapter Four glossary

choice – the correct answer

distractors – incorrect answers

mind palace – a way to create a visual memory space

mnemonics – a memory technique that uses the first letter of chosen words to create a new sentence or rhyme that is easy to recall

stem – the 'question' part of an MCQ question

units – for numerical information – mg / ml / % / kg / l / g, etc.

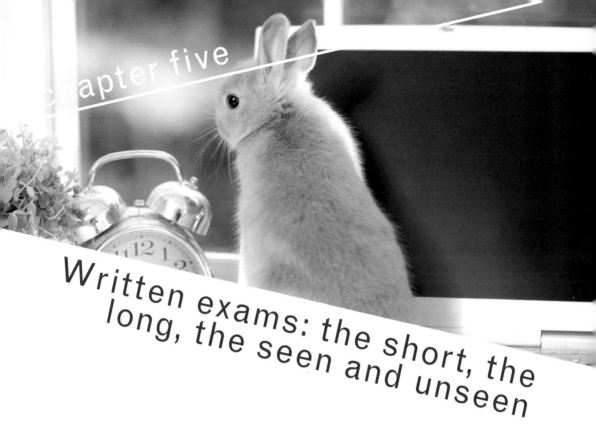

Written exams: the short, the long, the seen and unseen

Written exams may not hold the same fear factor as MCQ exams but they are still exams, and require you to prove your knowledge. While some people feel they are easier than an MCQ exam they are not necessarily any easier, they just require different skills.

Planning your revision

At this early point, I think it is a good time to introduce the fabulous Exam Prep Checklist from Stella Cottrell (Cottrell, 2013). It is a great starting point for revision for all exams but it is a particularly good guide for what you need to know about your written exam.

The original 17 steps are Cottrell's and I have added some extra information and created a table for you to use. It is important to note that you will not be able to complete all 17 steps when you start your revision. That is why I have created the table so you can plan when to tackle each of these steps. Some will be completed on the first day of a new module or a new term, when you get exam

Table 5.1 Exam prep checklist (adapted from Cottrell, 2013)

	Exam checklist	Yes	Date planned	Yes
1	I know exactly when the exams are			
	Dates, times, places			
2	I am aware how many questions are required for each exam			
	• Format of exam			
3	I have read the course or module details carefully to check what I am expected to know about the subject			
	• Make this your revision starting point			
	• Review the learning outcomes for the area to be assessed			
4	I have organized my notes so that the material is easy to learn			
	As per previous chapters this should be an ongoing process. Colour coding folders does not count as revision			
5	I can find something positive for me in taking these exams			
	One step closer to qualification			
6	I can develop the right frame of mind for these exams			
	Encourage yourself to study rather than force yourself			
7	I can work out how many topics I need to revise for each exam			
	• From points 4 and 5			
8	I am aware of the range of questions that can come up for each topic			
9	I have made a realistic revision timetable, with clear priorities			
	• Be honest with yourself about your responsibilities, time available, learning speed and stamina			
10	I know how to work on exam answers using past papers			
	• Especially important for writing skills			
11	I have started to practise writing out answers at speed			
	• Time your attempts at past papers and at your own revision questions			
12	I am aware of the memory strategies I need to revise for the exam			
	• Review Chapter Four for memory aides and find the style that suits you best			
13	I know how the marks are weighted for each question			
	• Helps select which questions to answer first			

Exam checklist	Yes	Date planned	Yes
14 I am aware of how to use time most effectively in the exam			
• Reading questions, planning answers and playing to your strengths			
15 I am aware of how to avoid common pitfalls in exams			
• Know your own pitfalls			
16 I am aware of the differences between exam answers and course work			
• Referencing and citations			
17 I know how to manage stress and use it effectively			
• Turning exam nerves into positive energy			

dates, times, location and format. Other steps will take time to work through, such as reading the course work, practising writing answers and finding good memory strategies.

> 'You cannot change what you are, only what you do.'
> – Philip Pullman, The Golden Compass

Once you have your revision plan in place what could go wrong? With **short-** and **long-answer questions** there is plenty of scope to write what you know and gain a few marks and not disgrace yourself? Isn't there?

In some senses that is correct. However, as we discussed in Chapter Four you are more likely to gain higher marks in MCQ exams. What can you do to try and gain high marks in written exams?

Revising for written exams

Much of what is written here applies to any exam. Much of it is common sense and I imagine you have heard it before. Nonetheless, as you progress on your academic journey you may find your needs change so it is worth reviewing how you prepare for exams regularly.

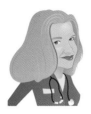

Caffeine fuelled all-night sessions may seem to be the road to success but they rarely are.

There will be times when you have multiple deadlines and responsibilities outside your course and you will feel an all-night session may be the best way forward. However, it is not the most sensible option and should be avoided if at all possible.

Keep yourself healthy and happy. Eat well, sleep well. Have a schedule and make time for something you enjoy. Even if you do not usually make some time for exercise, a simple 20-minute walk daily boosts your feeling of well-being, gets you away from your desk and can help you sleep better. It is free and good for you – what is not to like?

You should also be realistic about what you can cope with outside your college work. There will be times where you will need to say, 'No', to friends and family to prioritize your work. This can be very hard to do, so make sure if you sacrifice family and friend time that you make the best use of the time studying.

Revision is best in short sessions split up with breaks and rewards, and different activities. Remember Chapter One and the approaches to learning we looked at? Head back there to refresh your memory on planning, diaries and finding study plans that work for you. Keep your revision as interesting as possible. As mentioned in Chapter Four our brain works better at remembering when it is relaxed and enjoying itself. By planning breaks and rewards you keep it fun. Use the memory aides from Chapter Four to help bring something different and personal for you, remember Cottrell in Chapter One – be creative!

Not all subjects on your course will be as interesting to you as others. Some you will find harder than others. However, you need to pass these too. Be prepared to spend a little longer on areas you do not enjoy, as it may take longer to work through the material.

Be honest with yourself about what you need to achieve, it is the only way to succeed. Revision is personal to you. While studying in a group may be good for motivation, what you are each doing needs to reflect your own needs.

One good option is to meet to review material together, but then to learn that material by yourself, in your way.

With regard to exam revision you will hopefully have ready your course notes and access to reading lists and module information. If you do not – do not panic, you can still succeed. You will just have to work a bit faster and harder. Making notes as your course progresses and reviewing lecture notes during term time is the best way to avoid last minute scrabbles to collect and organize your research.

You are more likely to retain information you have read more than once. In an ideal world, information from taught sessions will have been accessed at least four times before you start revising for exams. This sounds like a hard challenge but it is possible, without spending your whole life in studying.

> 'Hope holds you fast like an anchor so you don't give way.'
> – Philip Pullman, The Golden Compass

Ideally you will have:

- carried out pre-lecture reading
- attended the lecture and made notes
- reviewed those notes post lecture
- checked any new terminology, or areas where your knowledge was lacking.

Pre-revision information gathering

The checklist below is not exhaustive but covers the basics of what you need to do *before* the studying begins:

- pre-revision information checking
- check subject area
- check exam requirements – what are the learning outcomes
- compile your notes and resources for the exam subject area
- lecture/seminar notes – ensure they are in the correct order.

You will then start your revision feeling that you a good command of the notes you have made and can make connections across the information you have.

Revision for an exam is different to preparing for an assignment, it can feel odd preparing for an exam after having written so many assignments. You do not need to have reference, so your revision can be more focused on a smaller set of resources that you understand well, can recall and in which you can identify the themes and arguments easily.

Therefore, there should be less time spent on research when preparing for exams. While you may need to read around the subject a little more to fill any gaps in knowledge you feel you have, the small depth is not required as for a 3000-word assignment.

Head back to Chapter One to check the learning styles and note making skills, and make use of this chapter's exam planning downloads. Now let us head on to how to approach a long- and short-answer exam.

Reading questions accurately

As with MCQ exams this is really important. The best advice is to read any questions twice before you decide what to do. Some books advise underlining or highlighting key words in the question. This may be harder to do in an online exam but you can write down questions and then read and annotate them if that is easier.

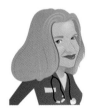

Don't be afraid to do things in your own style to help you succeed.

When reading the question try to spot the words that guide you to what the examiner wants you to answer. We can sometimes read exam questions and see the question we want to see rather than the question that is there.

There are a number of words that will be used to demonstrate to you what the examiner is looking for. There are numerous guides to these key verbs on the internet but I think the University of Kent has the simplest two-page guide. The full document is online, and some of the question types may not appear in a vet nursing course – this document is for all university courses, and also for all assessment types. To help you I have summarized in Table 5.2 the most likely options for vet nursing written exams, and these can also help you understand the wording of learning outcomes too. Identifying the key verbs and knowing what they mean will help you answer questions correctly, saving time and allowing you to progress through the exam paper.

Table 5.2 Exam words – examples (adapted from University of Kent, 2008)

Account for

Give reasons for; explain (note: give an account of = describe)

e.g. Account for the difference between female cat and dog reproductive cycles

Analyse

Break the information into constituent parts; examine the relationship between the parts; question the information

e.g. Analyse the management of stress in cats and dogs in the veterinary hospital

Clarify

Identify the components of an issue/topic/problem/; make the meaning plain; remove misunderstandings

e.g. Clarify the benefits of early neutering in cats

Compare

Look for similarities and differences between; perhaps conclude which is preferable; implies evaluation

e.g. Compare the anatomy and physiology of the hindlimbs of the canine and equine species

Contrast

Bring out the differences

e.g. Contrast the duties that can legally be undertaken by lay staff, SVNs and RVNs

Define

Give the precise meaning

e.g. Define the role of angiotensin in feline hypertension

Describe

Give a detailed, full account of the topic

e.g. Describe the process for gaining informed consent from a client

Discuss

Investigate or examine by argument; debate; give reason for and against; examine the implications of the topic

e.g. Discuss the nutritional issues of feeding a vegetarian diet to a dog

Table 5.2 continued

Evaluate/weigh up

Appraise the worth of something in the light of its truth or usefulness; assess and explain

e.g. Evaluate the role of weight management in the prevention and treatment of canine arthritis

Explain

Make plain and clear; give reasons for

e.g. Explain the care of an intravenous catheter in the feline patient

Identify

Point out and describe - trends/patterns/changes/ movements in certain directions (e.g. over time or across topics/ subjects)

e.g. Identify the changing role of the vet nurse from the inception of the title in 1984

Outline

Give a short description of the main points; give the main features or general principles; emphasize the structure

e.g. Outline the changes to the cardiovascular system in a dog with DCM

Summarize

Give a concise account of the chief points of a matter, removing unnecessary detail

e.g. summarize the nursing care required for splint bandages in a dog

How exam questions are set

While the key verbs can be used at different levels of academic writing you need to ensure you are answering at the level required. If you include too much basic information

> 'All the history of human life has been a struggle between wisdom and stupidity.'
> – Philip Pullman, The Amber Spyglass

you will waste time providing information that will not gain you higher marks and may use up time that you could have better used to gain marks in other questions. Consider if what you have written as an answer would be suitable for the level required. While you may think that you do not understand the differences between the levels of academic courses you can set your own standards to check what you are writing.

Consider the exam question and decide if your answer could be used to describe the information to a client or friend, a fellow SVN, an experienced RVN or vet, or published in an academic journal. You will be able to move towards more academic writing by:

- using appropriate terminology
- informally referencing answers by using surnames of authors of relevant work.

Do not waste time with long winded answers, keep it succinct.

Keeping these points in mind, then consider the question type. If the question asks you to 'describe' it means just that – describe something. There is no need to start analysing or critiquing what you have been asked to describe.

There will be a variety of verbs used. As you have probably realized, these ask you to display differing levels of knowledge. There is a straightforward 'describe' but also the more in depth 'contrast' or 'analyse'. With these questions, you are moving on from descriptions of what you know and demonstrating understanding of knowledge as well as the ability to recall it.

With questions that ask for analysis or ask you to contrast/compare information be careful not to fall into the trap of thinking you have answered it well just by writing a lot – these question types need more than descriptive paragraphs. Make sure you work to address all the major points from the question and limit descriptive passages to setting up the point you are trying to make.

You will also be guided on how much you need to write by the marks given for each question, use these to guide you on the time to spend on each question and on the amount of detail you need to go into on each question.

Imagine you are faced with two questions in the first section of an exam – both worth 10 marks each. One subject you are very confident on, the second you are less confident on. Which question do you spend most time on?

Sorry, this is a bit of a trick question. If you are confident in answering a question then it should take you less time than a question you are less confident on. You also do not want to spend longer than needed on the question you are less confident on. There may be other questions that you will be confident on in later sections, so do not get bogged down pouring everything into the first question you read or battling with an early question you are struggling with.

Planning your time in the exam

This means putting all the above into practice and making sure that you read through the exam paper in full before you start writing. This might seem to be not a good use of your time, but it is essential in ensuring you spend the correct amount of time on each question and at the outset identify the questions you may struggle with.

> **Read ALL the questions BEFORE you answer them.**

Once you have read the questions you need to identify:

- what they are asking
- which you are most confident answering
- how much those questions are worth
- how much time to devote to each question.

I would advise using the start of a written exam to work through this plan. Then jot down each question number and how long you will spend on it – and stick to that. Do not get side tracked by writing a fabulous answer showing everything you know on the endocrine system when the question is only worth four marks.

Work through each question and answer them all. You cannot gain marks if you have not written an answer, even if you are unsure about the question write down what you can to answer the question. I repeat, do not fall into the trap of throwing down everything you have ever heard about the subject – stick to answering what is asked. Your answer will be succinct, will not have taken much time and may still gain higher marks.

> '*When you choose one way out of many, all the ways you don't take are snuffed out like candles, as if they'd never existed.*'
> – Philip Pullman, The Amber Spyglass

Remember that the examiner can only give you the maximum amount of marks there are available for a question. Writing excessively on your favourite areas will only use up time and not guarantee higher marks.

You do have time to plan your answer

It is worth jotting down the basic points you wish to cover – if it is a computer-based exam use the paper provided for note making to do this. A short plan, even of only four or five bullet points will ensure that as you expand on each point you do not spend too long on it and forget what else you wanted to say. Making a 'notes' section also allows you to write down any memory aides you have to recall.

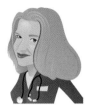

> *Give yourself time and space to achieve in your exam.*

You should aim to write a focused a mini-essay. Although a long paragraph for an introduction is too much it can help to repeat the question, or paraphrase it when you start your answer. This helps focus your mind on what you want to say and confirms to the examiner that you have read and understood the exam question. It can also set your answer up nicely for using bullet points or short statements rather than launching into long-winded paragraphs. Bullet points are acceptable in written answers as long as they are used correctly, to show a lot of information in a small space and to start a longer discussion of these points in a limited time situation such as an exam. However, you may find you get lower marks if you simply provide a bullet point list or use only this way to present information. There is still space for a conclusion. Again, avoid a long paragraph and focus on showing you have answered the question asked in a few sentences.

Getting across ideas, opinions and theories

How to answer a short- or long-answer question

This might seem a question to which you already know the answer. You already write assignments and have sat written exams before starting this course. What else could there be to know?

This does not mean you can become too relaxed but you can worry less about spelling and grammar and punctuation. You should still try to present your work well, but the occasional typo or grammatical error will not lose marks as it would in an assignment. As long as it is clear to the examiner what you mean then you should not lose marks for poor presentation.

While it can be liberating to write without the need for full referencing it can make you think you do not need to discuss ideas and arguments that you would need to reference in an assignment. But you can. In fact, you should in questions asking for analysis or comparison.

You can informally reference works you have read during your course. No need for full Harvard style, but stating surnames and years of publication (if possible) in your answer are enough. It demonstrates

> An exam is different from an assignment.

you are clear about what are your own views and which are views informed by others work. If certain works have helped you then stating the surname of the author and relating it to your answer is helpful and shows what you have read. Any quotes do not have to be exact and you can paraphrase them.

The exam is testing your knowledge and skills learned from the course. You have been assessed on your ability to research and demonstrate using the research of others to inform your knowledge. An exam is looking for your experience of the course material and how you understood it. Examiners will be impressed if you do more than just regurgitate the course notes.

In contrast to MCQ exams, written exams are less about recalling content and more about your ideas and confirming what you have learned. While you can answer many exam questions by recalling course notes you will gain better marks in the tougher questions, which ask you to analyse or critique information or ideas, if you have spent less time memorizing facts and more time on ideas and concepts backed up by course material.

Calculations and numerical data

In a written exam, you may be given information to appraise and discuss. This removes the need to describe information and you need to be able to show an analysis of the information. While you could be given a case study of a client or patient, you may also be given statistical or numerical data. This can scare some people, even if there are no calculations involved. We use numeracy skills every day in practice, yet many people find numerical data stressful.

> *Questions with calculations are not there to catch you out, but to show that you can do what you need to do in work every day.*

You may be given numerical evidence to review and analyse in your exam, or you may be given calculations to work out. Unless you are informed otherwise you will be provided with a calculator. Return to Chapter Four for more on calculations in exams.

Facts and figures

In both pre- and post-qualification courses you may be given numerical data to analyse. Do not be scared. It sounds worse than it is, it is very similar to being asked to analyse written data.

Reading numerical information is a skill you already have – you check prices on items before you buy them, you have probably used comparison websites to check prices and information on products from holidays to pet insurance. Reading numerical information in an exam is very similar.

Tables, graphs and pie charts are all simple ways to show numerical data. There are advantages and disadvantages to all ways of showing data. To help you read the data quickly and easily here are a few tips:

- read the title of the information given, and the information on the axes
- take your time and read slowly and clearly
- scan the values for highs, lows and any 'outliers' (numbers that do not fit the pattern or that you do not expect – for example, a factor of 0 for a PCV)
- make notes of interesting points – low scores or unexpected data
- check for the source of the data.

These tips will help you see what the data is telling you and make it easier to check facts and information.

Compare the two charts in Figures 5.1 and 5.2. Although they are for different information, from reading the information given about the data provided, which is the most reliable? Use the points above to make your own notes and then see if this matches my summaries.

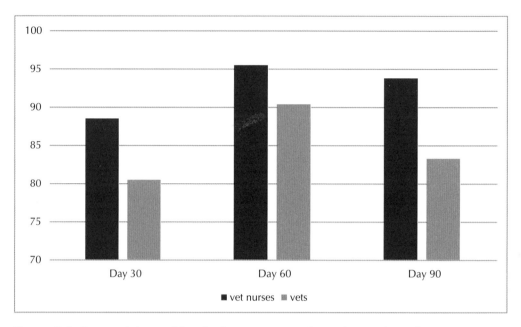

Figure 5.1 Successful searching for lost otoscopes from day 0 of employment

Figure 5.1 summary:

- consistently high data figures provided
- low 80%
- high 95%
- axis % on one side and period of trial on the other
- timescale limited to 90 days
- two coloured columns – one for vets and one for vet nurses
- no number of how many involved in research – how much is 100%?
- no comparison with other staff, or any training differences that may affect results
- data from a company that supports vet nurses – is this data bias?

Figure 5.2 summary:

- varied data
- gradual decline overall
- high – 6500 neuters but over a year or a decade?
- low less than 2000 but again no time frame

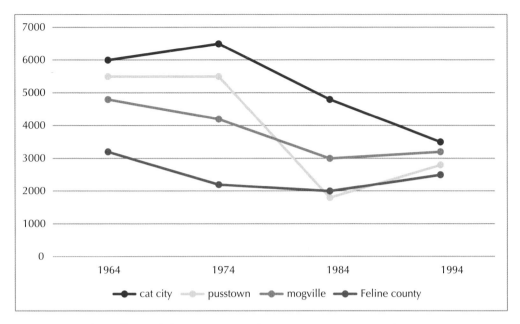

Figure 5.2 The effect of the 1974 mandatory cat neutering scheme on neutering numbers in 4 towns in the UK

- timescale 1964–1994
- information on axes not clear – is the time frame a year of each decade or total for each decade?
- no idea on how large the towns are so no idea of the percentage of cats of the total population are neutered
- no reference to source of data (government data or charities or a mix?)
- has the mandatory neutering scheme worked in terms of trends or overall numbers neutered?

These are a very basic quick summary of the two figures, using the tips above:

- read the information
- note highs and lows
- note outlying information or anomalies (introduction of mandatory neutering)
- note where the information is coming from or any biased reporting.

You can see that in a short space of time you have a much clearer view on the validity of the information and any data that is interesting or unusual. It is an easier way to scan the information than reading each line or bar individually.

It may be worth reviewing this information if you are going to use statistics and data analysis in your own research – as discussed in a dissertation in Chapter Three.

Understanding numerical terms

- Mean – average
- Median – middle of the range of figures
- Mode – the one that appears most frequently
- Range – the difference between highest and lowest

You could be asked to comment on these. You might recall them from school maths exams but you might not remember them now. Head back to Chapter Three for more information on statistical analysis.

Open book/seen exams

It is now a good time to mention **open book/seen exams**, similar to MCQ exams some people can approach these with little preparation assuming all the answers will be in front of them – yes?

Well, similar to MCQs there is still a need to prepare. Open book exams are used to show you have an understanding of a subject and also are aware of resources to use. They are especially useful as an assessment tool in areas where information may change so you need to check resources regularly, they are a way to assess how you work with information resources.

In an open book exam you are advised of the resources you will have in the exam but not the questions or scenarios you are required to address. In this style of exam, you are asked to present information and evidence from the given texts to support your answers. The length or structure of your answer is less important than demonstrating you know how the information in the texts given apply to the answers you provide.

In a seen exam, the questions are provided in advance so you can research but you cannot take notes or resources into the exam. The purpose of this style of exam is to allow you to research and create a more in depth and structured answer than you would normally be able to produce in an unseen exam.

Both work in different ways and both require preparation, do not be fooled with either that you can do less preparation work than for other exam types – is just different preparation.

For both you are given some extra information in advance – make sure you make time to use that information. For open book exams make sure you are familiar with the layout of the texts and where you will find information for the exam subject area. Outside of veterinary nursing they are used in subject areas where you may need to make accurate references to data, including numerical data, or to specific legislation so they are often used for law or accountancy or economics exams.

For both types of assessment, you still need to plan time to prepare and understand the subject area and assessment type. Head to Chapter One to check the planning and organization tips and Chapter Two for research skills and accessing information.

Typing or writing?

This might seem an unusual question as you do not have a choice in the way the exam is set up, but make sure you know the medium the exam will use and prepare for it too.

Today many exams are set on computers. As most students now have had an education centred around using computers this seems to be normal. For mature students, this might be an added hurdle to achieve – as the computers and the software used in education might be less familiar. We also use touch screen devices more often than sitting at a desktop and typing, so even those that think they use 'computers' a lot are using phones and tablets.

You may wish to consider your learning needs in terms of the medium of the exam. Check the learning needs section in Chapter One and consider if you are hindered by the way the exam is set and whether can you make any reasonable changes to help you – pen types, coloured overlays for screen or exam scripts – it's worth speaking to your

> *The medium in which the exam is set may affect your ability to recall and set down information.*

course provider if you have any concerns. With my noted mobility issues, I have been allowed to sit written exams in separate rooms so I can stretch and move around without disturbing other exam takers.

There are ways to help everyone succeed with typed exams. You may also find some of these techniques improve your note making and study skills too!

Touch typing

Not just for admin types. This is a longer-term plan so do not attempt it the week before an exam – if you do not already touch type then plan to learn when you have a lighter workload. There are numerous benefits. You cannot touch type with poor posture, you have to sit well and this reduces the strain on your back and other joints. You will produce fewer mistakes when typing and the process will be less frustrating.

You will get better and faster the more you do it, and it makes tackling larger assignments less stressful. You also watch the screen and see what you are creating and that helps the flow of writing. Otherwise you tend to tap out a sentence and then check it on the screen, correcting typos and mistakes at the time. This slows down your train of thought and may interrupt some great ideas. This is often why people prefer to make notes and start essays with pen and paper – to let their ideas flow.

You can achieve this flow with typing, you just need to get over the hurdle of typing efficiently first – it took me a while but I managed it and have found it really useful in reducing the time it takes me to write.

Posture

As above – it is so important to be comfortable when writing in an exam. Check how you sit when typing – is it comfortable? Can you maintain that posture for 30–60 minutes without getting up? If the answer is No, then do consider checking out some resources for sitting comfortably at a desk. You will need to re-adjust your seating position in exams so consider how to do that comfortably, safely and without knocking your notes and pens to the floor. I like gentle head rolls from side to side, gentle breathing and some shoulder rolls backwards and forwards. Also consider your feet – are they flat on the floor and able to support your weight evenly? Crossing your legs can feel natural but it is not a position you can sustain comfortably for an extended period.

Practice

Yes, more practice. This time practice how you will write your exam answers. Not just the content and the layout but the typing or writing required. If you only type for the final draft of an assignment then you will not be comfortable typing at speed while processing your thoughts in an exam. It's another non-academic skill that can help you succeed.

Using written aides in an exam

While you cannot take written aides in to an unseen exam you can create them once you are in the exam. You will always be given paper and pen in an exam. This is to allow you to write down calculations, or notes, or work out answers. Use this to your advantage if you prefer writing to typing. As I have mentioned before, do not be afraid to make your own little notes in an exam – even before you view the questions. If you have some memory aides to help you then write them down, the same with calculations.

As mentioned above, make use of the paper and turn it into a revision sheet. This reduces stress as it reduces the number of things you feel you need to remember at the start of an exam. You can also use the paper to plan your exam and your answers. Keep a tick box for each question answered so you know you have completed the exam according to the instructions.

> 'We shouldn't live as if [other worlds] mattered more than this life in this world, because where we are is always the most important place.'
> – Philip Pullman, The Amber Spyglass

On the day

I have encountered students who feel that revising hard for exams is pointless as their inability to perform well on exam day means they cannot show how much work they have done or how much they know. This leads to a negative cycle of less revision, nerves and poor exam performances.

Read Chapter One on exam nerves and consider how you can improve your personal ability to remain calm and be able to give the exam your best effort. Prepare as best you can, plan and manage your time to stop the feelings of doubt setting in and affecting your plans. Check the exam prep checklist provide above.

> *Breathe.*
> *Focus on the immediate question.*
> *Do what is asked of you.*

Before you head over to check what to do on the day of the exam, remember that it is just an exam, you have got this far and you can do well.

 Review Chapter 5 and how to apply what you have learned with the Reflective Template.

Chapter Five glossary

Long-answer questions – exam questions requiring answers structured like a short essay

Open book exam – an exam where you are permitted to take in set texts or a set amount of notes

Seen exam – an exam where you are allowed access to the questions prior to the exam

Short-answer questions – exam questions requiring bullet point or answers around a paragraph long

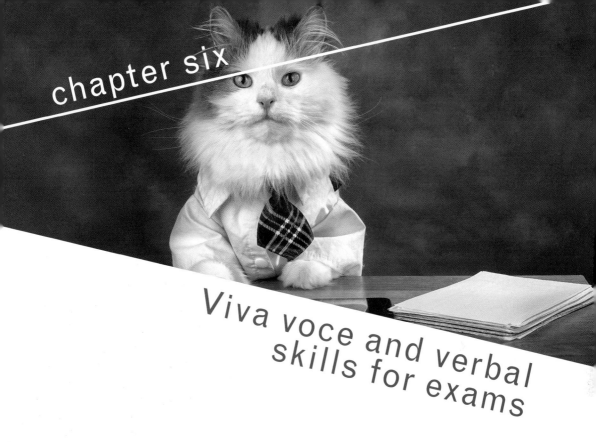

chapter six

Viva voce and verbal skills for exams

While the use of viva voce exams is limited in vet nursing undergraduate programmes they are often used in more advanced qualifications and even if you do not have to face one now, the skills required can help in many other situations. Being confident when talking face to face with an examiner can help you in OSCE exams, during your work-based learning and for job interviews.

Viva exams are used more commonly in post-graduate qualifications and as there are now master's courses available in vet nursing and also doctorates in associated fields they will become more common.

Spoken assessments feature in case-based discussions and chart-stimulated recall exams. As vet nursing assessment progresses with work-based assessments the overlap between traditional viva exams and the use of these types of examinations may well increase.

'Don't gobblefunk around with words.'
– Roald Dahl, The BFG

What are they?

A viva voce is commonly referred to as a viva and is a spoken exam. I am being careful not to say **oral exam** as although this is the term sometimes used it more usually refers to exams taken by language students to demonstrate their level of competency in a foreign language. The phrase 'viva voce' simply means 'living voice' or 'by word of mouth'.

A spoken exam is where the examiner or examiners ask verbal questions regarding your work and you discuss various aspects of your knowledge. Do not be surprised if you have two examiners, it is common practice to have an examiner and an observer, or a lead examiner and support examiner. This is from a safety and standardization of exams point of view and is normal; do not let the audience size put you off!

Spoken exam nerves can be daunting and many people find that nerves affect how they perform. While we have already covered some aspects of dealing with exam nerves there are some specific tips for spoken and practical exams, and there is more on practical exams in Chapter Seven.

We can all get tongue tied and feel we cannot say what we mean. That is perfectly normal in an exam. I would advise to start simply, and in response to a question start working with what enters your head. There is no point trying to formulate a long answer that says everything about your work straight away. The examiners are not expecting that, and answering the question asked is enough and the examiners can prompt you to say more.

What do they assess?

For many educational institutions, the viva is to prove ownership of a student's written work through discussing the thought process around the project and is a chance to allow the student to discuss their research and the supporting information. Questions will be used to explore your feelings and thoughts around what you researched and why you chose this subject area. Your research methods and results will be questioned.

Vivas can also assess ethical issues, professional issues and communication skills. For instance, in human medicine they are used along with OSCEs to assess patient–doctor communication, to give you an idea of their uses in other fields.

There are two commonly used areas for viva exams:

- to assess the knowledge gained from writing an extended piece of work, such as a dissertation
- to provide further information where there are borderline marks between grades that can affect the overall degree grading.

They may also be used as part of a college or university's academic process and you may be asked to attend one in the following circumstances, as:

- an interview rather than an exam to assess academic standards (this type of discussion has no bearing on an individual's mark)
- part of an investigation into suspected plagiarism or fraudulent submissions of work.

Spoken exams are a way of showing you have the knowledge to have produced the work you submitted. It provides an opportunity to 'show how' when you have already completed the 'does' aspect of **Miller's Pyramid of Knowledge** (Figure 6.1).

Showing that you know how to do something is important in science courses as there is always a practical element to the course with lab work, and in vet nursing clinical skills are assessed via practical exams and the viva shows you have the ability to research and apply the knowledge gained to your working life.

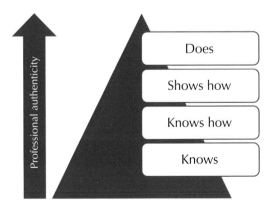

Figure 6.1 A model of competence (adapted from the Miller's [1990] Pyramid of Knowledge)

'If you have good thoughts they will shine out of your face like sunbeams and you will always look lovely.'
– Roald Dahl, The Twits

It is important to note that a viva is *not* assessing your ability to speak in public. While speaking clearly and coherently is expected, if you pause or take time to think, that will not be marked against you.

It is most likely you will sit a viva as part of the assessment of your extended writing, where it is a planned part of your assessment. This gives you time to plan and prepare.

How to prepare

Preparation is similar to other exams, you need to know your work on the subject area thoroughly, but you also need to know about the process you went through in researching your work, how you found the information that formed your opinions and what were the main influences. If this was a piece of original research then the data collated and reviewed, and the methods used will also be important so you should be prepared to discuss these. This will include the way you have interpreted the data and possible implications for future research.

Making notes on your subject area is still a great place to start, as is finding out about common questions and practising potential answers.

Making your notes 'speak'

While it can feel counterintuitive you can use your notes and turn them into a narrative for a speech or as a short passage for the answer to a question in a viva exam. Return to Chapter One for advice on making notes for revision, and Chapter Nine for notes on public speaking.

Take the relevant notes you have made and turn them either into a speech or answers to possible questions. It can help to pose questions to yourself and answer them with the notes you have made and see if they make sense. This may also help you write in a way that is easier to practise saying aloud and will feel more natural in the exam.

Reading work aloud also helps you see if your writing flows and if there are any gaps in the information. While it can feel nerve wracking reading aloud to others, once you are comfortable with your work, reading it to someone else – even someone with little or no knowledge of your subject – can be really helpful. It can help you start to work at controlling your nerves and improve your exam **presentation** skills.

Practising

You will be addressing your answers to an examiner and possibly an assistant examiner, which is a little different to any practical exams/OSCEs you may have taken where the examiner tries to be an unobtrusive observer. Practising with other people is not the first thing you should attempt, it will not feel natural at first, but once you are at the stage of re-reading notes it is time to try reading them aloud and then to read them to other people.

You may also benefit from asking yourself questions, rather like making your own MCQs to aid revision. Thinking of the information a viva examiner might want to know will help you form some questions to answer.

Practise viva questions

The following are commonly used viva questions, and expansions on what they mean and what you should consider including in your responses.

What is it about?

*   Summarize your written work, highlighting key areas and findings.

What did you do?

- How did you find the information, what research methods did you use and what influenced you?
- This is a time to give your opinions and feelings about the process and what you found out. Think about it as a more formal version of how you would talk about the experience with class mates.

What did you find?

- What was the result?
- What did the data show, how did you feel about this and how did this compare to what you thought at the start of the project?

Why does that matter?

- What are the future implications of your research? Is there a need for further research or more work on the area? What might change in the field in the near future?

The examiner wants you to do your best and knows you will do better when you feel comfortable. Therefore open, conversational questions are usually used at the start of the exam. Closed and more specific questions will be used once you have mentioned key areas and specific information and finding. Questions will cover areas in a similar pattern to the layout of an assignment: general information, research conducted, findings, discussion and conclusion. Making notes on these areas will create a great starting point for your answers.

'"Words," he said, "is oh such a twitch-tickling problem to me all my life."'
– Roald Dahl, The BFG

General questions

- Why did you choose this subject area?
- How did your thoughts on the subject change as you researched further?
- What were the most interesting or enjoyable aspects of the research?
- Did the research change the way you nurse?

Research conducted

- Who were the key authors or researchers that influenced your journey?
- What future research would benefit this area?
- You have not used X paper/author's work, which is widely read in this area, why is that?

Research methods

Questions here will focus on the **methodology** you used to find data and the way you interpreted this. Be prepared to talk about the way you chose your methodology and statistical interpretations as these are as important as the findings themselves.

Analysis and findings

- What were your ways of analysing data and how did this influence your findings?
- Did you expect these results, and if not, what did you expect?

All of these questions are leading you into a wider discussion on your work where there are less interventions from the examiners and you are given the opportunity to talk more freely about the project.

Discussion

This can feel like a relaxing part of the exam! But the discussion of how you felt about the process is very important so remember to keep it professional. You are likely to be asked reflective questions.

- Now the project is complete would you carry out the research and analysis in the same way if you had to do it again?
- What would you change about the project to improve it?
- Is there anything you definitely would not do again?

Conclusions/Implications

I will leave the final two questions to the University of Leicester's great advice on sitting a viva.

- What are the empirical, practice, and theoretical implications of your findings?
- How would you hope that this research could be followed up and taken further?

These questions can sound quite complicated but you will already have written about these implications in your work so try to summarize these areas and also refer to anything else you have said previously if it answers the question.

Viva exams are about being familiar with your work. Reading your work aloud will help you reflect on the decisions you made and be confident in speaking about your experiences. Reading your notes aloud will also let you establish prompts to help you remember what you wanted to say, even when you are nervous.

You can link to key words that will appear in your subject area and also focus on the way questions may be phrased. Questions may ask for your knowledge – what you know about

> 'It's impossible to make your eyes twinkle if you aren't feeling twinkly yourself.'
> – *Roald Dahl*, Danny, the Champion of the World

the subject – but also how you applied the knowledge and what your research methods were and how you chose them. This is particularly true for original research and using your data to predict what could happen in the future.

On the day

Check out the On The Day planner online and if you head back to Chapter Two there is more information about using notes from assignments and dissertations for revising for oral exams. Also have a look at the Exam Prep Checklist in Chapter Five.

Have a plan in your mind of the message you wish to get across in the viva. Yes, they will ask similar questions to all candidates, but this is your personal work so decide what you want to say about it. Use the key words

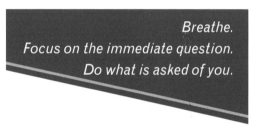

Breathe.
Focus on the immediate question.
Do what is asked of you.

as hooks to build answers around. Similar to the plan in Chapter Seven for OSCE exams have a 4–5 step plan for the exam or for likely questions. This will help you focus your thoughts and help keep nerves from making you too nervous.

Physical presence in a spoken exam

In my experience, one of the nice things about written exams is that even if you are not confident in what you have written it is unlikely you will ever meet the exam marker to explain what you wrote and why. With spoken exams you are verbalising your written words in a situation where people can ask you questions on your work. It is quite a stressful situation. Your physical presence in the exam can help you overcome nerves and help your performance.

Sitting comfortably

You are usually offered a chair in a viva and the examiners are usually seated too. Make use of the chair and sit fully on it supported by the back rest. This will allow you to relax a little and be comfortable.

Body language can be hard to get right when you are nervous. It is most important to be yourself as much as you can. If you usually gesture with your hands when talking, then continue to do so. Try to sit without crossing your legs or arms if you can, but other than that, be yourself.

What to wear

Try to dress as if attending a job interview. This does not mean going out to buy new clothes, but wearing the smartest clothes you have and ensuring they are clean and well presented. A suit or smart trousers/skirt with shirt or a smart dress are all acceptable. Remember to wear something that fits you and you feel comfortable in and which looks good when sitting down. Shorts, or short skirts might not be the best, even in warm weather as they may be considered too informal. Also consider neck lines: if your skin turns red when stressed consider higher necklines to cover this.

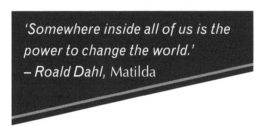

'Somewhere inside all of us is the power to change the world.'
– Roald Dahl, Matilda

Public speaking and presentations

While the viva is not used as much in undergraduate vet nurse education the skills and preparation described in this chapter can be used in other situations. It is likely that during your training you will be asked to present to your class mates or colleagues, and during your career as a vet nurse there are often situations where you need to speak to a group. Let us look at how you can use viva skills to improve your experiences of speaking to groups.

Knowledge

Make sure you really do know your subject area. When you are researching, if you have a question about what you are reading then the audience is likely to think the same. Find the answer to the questions you want answered and you will be well prepared. If people do ask something you are not 100% sure of then it is perfectly acceptable to say that you will check the details and get back to them – you are not expected to be the font of *all* knowledge on the subject.

Your audience: clients, school children, colleagues

You need to consider your audience and apply your knowledge appropriately. You may be talking to colleagues for CPD, to clients to share information or to school or college students about the role of a vet nurse.

Consider your audience in your delivery – especially the use of terminology and anatomical terms. We use these and acronyms easily every day but forget that this can sound like a different language to those not in the industry.

Note making

As above, make written or typed notes on what you are going to talk about. While some people can feel this might make them read directly from their notes, your presentation will be easier to recall with some short prompts than using a printed out version of it in full. You may find the advice on note making for public speaking in Chapter Nine helpful.

Practice and breathing

Even the most experienced public speaker practises. I promise! While some people make it look easy there are some basic guidelines than can help you.

First, it is worth practising your speech. It can help you find the right tone, to identify the words and areas you wish to add emphasis to and also to check your timing. This is where your notes and prompts come in handy as you can write your timings alongside the notes, which will help you keep to time without needing to keep checking a clock.

As with all exams breathing is super important, to control your nerves and in this case to project your voice. As I advise in Chapter Seven on OSCEs, you need to focus on your breathing. Top tips include:

- breathing from your abdomen/diaphragm
- taking a deep breath before your start speaking (a deep breath to be one where you inhale for 5 seconds and exhale for 5 seconds)
- making space for you to breathe during your presentation – use pictures or videos as **visual aids** that allow you time and space to breathe.

Props and learning materials

Most people use some sort of presentation software to create a visual aid. However, these can be quite dull, especially if they are just a copy of your notes. They are of use to show pictures or videos that support what you say, but try to avoid using them for a lot of text. If you need to put text up, use just the important points you want people to remember, not everything you are going to say.

Your font style should be one that is accessible to all so check dyslexia guidelines and guidelines for the visually impaired. Certain fonts work better and try to avoid underlining words – instead use bold, a change of colour (but remember visual impairment) or increase the font size.

Font size is also important – it can easily emphasize words and should match the words you are emphasizing with your speech. Font size needs to be large enough to be read easily so consider 26 pt and above.

Pictures and videos will need copyright clearance so do check before you use them, broadly speaking if someone else has created it you should be asking for the right to use before you share it with others, and make sure you credit their work to them.

There are copyright free resources on the internet for images. You may need to sign up to the provider but there is usually no charge for one off or only occasional use.

Alternatives to viva exams

Viva skills are also useful if you are assessed via case-based discussions or chart-recall tests. At the time of writing, these are not used in veterinary nursing but could be introduced as assessments of written work and also in work-based assessments, such as in the Nursing Progress Log (NPL).

Case-based discussion

A case-based discussion is similar to the professional discussions that were used in the UK under a previous vet nurse training scheme. Within a given case or scenario the student should role play or respond to questions or prompts from their training supervisor as if it were a real situation.

Chart-recall exams

These are used in human medical training in the USA and have been developed in UK training systems based on the use of chart-recall assessments from the USA and Canada. Chart-recall exams use hospital charts to show information that has already been gathered about a patient and thus the student steps into a simulation of a case and is expected to carry on with the treatment as required from the hospital chart.

They are a step on from our current OSCE exams and are useful exams that require some communication between student and examiner and so skills for speaking in an exam are required.

These alternatives to viva exams are shown to assess the wider aspect of student learning. I know that clinical skills/viva exams are not always popular and exploring different ways to assess what is needed in a professional course is important. It may help you realize how much is required of these types of exams if you understand the contexts and competencies they assess.

Four contexts:

- patient
- teamwork
- personal
- society.

Three **competency areas**:

- communication
- professional values
- personal development. (Wass et al., 2003)

> 'You'll never get anywhere if you go about what-iffing like that.'
> – *Roald Dahl*, Charlie and the Great Glass Elevator

As the vet nurse role expands it is likely we will see exams of this style especially in post-qualification assessments.

 Review Chapter 6 and how to apply what you have learned with the Reflective Template.

Chapter Six glossary

competency areas – defined areas of clinical skills where competency needs to be confirmed

methodology – system of methods used to research a subject area

Miller's Pyramid of Knowledge – a system of assessing clinical competence

oral exam – language competence exams

presentation – the written part of a spoken presentation

visual aid – anything used to support a talk or lecture

viva voce – spoken exam

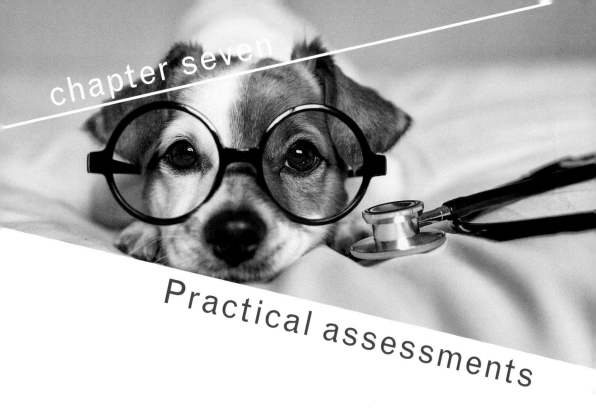

Practical assessments

There a number of ways the practical aspect of a vet nursing course is assessed, through work-based assessments and exams, which can take many different formats.

For exams, the **OSCE** is still the most common exam in the UK and it is used in many other countries. It is a reliable way to assess clinical skills and can be adapted to many medical specialisms, vet nursing included.

A combination of work-based assessment and exam via direct observation (DOPs) or case-based studies are becoming more common as an alternative to OSCEs. I will discuss the future options for clinical assessment at the end of this chapter, but I will start by looking at preparing for the standard OSCEs and this information can easily be applied to other **practical exams**.

What are OSCEs?

OSCEs are Objective Structured Clinical Exams. They are used in many areas and are very common in the medical field, you will not be alone in sitting these exams and there is a lot of research to support their use. They were developed in the 1970s by a human doctor and have been used ever since. They are an accurate and objective way to examine clinical skills. The idea behind them was to provide a way to examine clinical skills that would be fair to everyone and they do achieve this even though this is a hard thing to do. OSCE exams are a set of a minimum of 12 stations in one exam.

Some UK vet nursing degree programmes run practical exams at the end of associated modules and so may not choose to do 12 tasks on the same subject. Therefore, although the set-up of individual tasks is similar, they are called practical exams rather than OSCEs.

The areas examined by OSCEs or practical exams may vary but they usually focus on skills across clinical areas such as:

- in-patient work, such as preparing and administering medication
- anaesthesia skills
- theatre preparation skills
- diagnostics such as lab or imaging skills.

They were originally unique as exams as they provided a checklist of skills that a candidate needed to demonstrate to be able to pass the exam. Although these checklists were mainly written for the examiner and to allow feedback, they are now widely used by students as 'pass sheets' or as a definitive 'answer sheet'. We will consider later in this chapter if these are as helpful as you think!

Why are they used?

Assessing practical skills in veterinary medicine has always been difficult. Being able to assess skills in formal exams, such as OSCEs, provides a quality assurance aspect to the work-based assessments used in the UK via the Nursing Progress Log (NPL) or Clinical Skills Log (CSL).

There is a need to produce vet nurses that have the basic skills from the first day they qualify to carry out their **Day One Skills** in the UK, Veterinary Technology Student **Essential and Recommended Skills** list for the AVMA in the USA and meet the **Competency Standards** for the VNCA in Australia. Assessing practical skills properly is key to this.

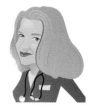

Despite what many people say they are not a 'box ticking' exercise.

The assessment of clinical skills is one reason the UK vet nursing education programme is so highly regarded. The stringent requirements of UK vet nursing education are also the reason there is not automatic entry onto the UK register for overseas vet nurses, many need to sit the pre-registration OSCEs from the Royal College of Veterinary Surgeons. This chapter can help people sitting these exams too.

OSCE myths

Of all exams, it seems that OSCEs cause the most stress. This is understandable, they are often the final exams standing between candidate vet nurses and qualification, and for many students they will need to go to an external exam centre, which can add to the stress. I have also found that the many myths surrounding OSCEs can add to the stress.

There are tales of evil examiners, students weeping, and of unusual or malfunctioning equipment. Over the years many tales have been shared and with each telling they become more real. I have found when teaching clinical skills that you need to battle through the built-up panic surrounding the myths before you can get to teaching the facts. Let us get through some of these myths and stop them becoming an unnecessary impediment to your preparation.

Examiners

All the examiners you meet are vets or RVNs. They are all experienced clinical coaches and have been trained to be examiners, they do not just arrive and pick up a clipboard and look for mistakes, they are there to help you pass. However, I know some students feel they are a little cold or stand-offish.

This is because examiners are limited in what they can say to students. Each student, pass or fail, first student of the day or last, must receive the same experience from the examiner. There can be no indication of how well the student has done in the exam, no extra smiles for passing or sad faces for a fail.

This means examiners cannot give any feedback during the exam process, and they cannot give information that would advantage any one student over the others. This really limits what they can say. You will often find their response is 'thank you'.

Contrary to popular belief you can ask questions of an examiner. However, to get the best response you need to ask direct questions. An open question, such as 'Is this ok?', is not going to get a response that helps you, but a direct question 'Where is the "On" switch for the microscope please?', can be answered. This is not information that will advantage you over another student. The examiner does not want you to waste time finding a switch, when this is not a demonstration of your clinical skills.

The exam is not titled 'On switches of microscopes, 1984–1992. 'If in doubt about something then ask the examiner. The worst they can say would be 'I can't answer that', but you have acknowledged your issue and will find it easier to move on than if you were silently worrying.

Examiners want to see you pass. There is nothing worse than watching a student complete a task but knowing they have not passed. They want you all to pass!

Venue

If you need to go to an external exam centre to attend your OSCEs it can add additional stress: not least finding it and adapting to the unusual surroundings. OSCE centres are not chosen to add to the stress. They are chosen for space, access to equipment, availability of examiners and resources, and yes, to try to offer an even spread of locations. When I qualified there were, I think, three OSCE centres across the whole of the UK, and the exams were held once a year. A long time to wait for a re-sit!

The provision of exam centres is limited, something exam providers are aware of, and there are many demands on the exam space. Venues need to have a large enough space to take a number of stations. That is a lot of space. They also need to be free for regular periods across the year. They also need to have some of the large equipment available or very close by. OSCE exams are expensive to set up and run. If the cost of moving large equipment was added, it would make the exams even more expensive, something all exam providers are aware of and try to avoid.

If you are worried about attending a different centre then see if they run OSCE revision days that you could attend, which will allow you to get to know the centre and how to get there. If they do not then check your travel routes well in advance and consider the most stress-free option for attending. Could an overnight stay be easier than travelling on the same day?

Equipment

While there are different centres for all OSCEs, from university courses to diploma the equipment used is standardized. It is not set to challenge you, it is equipment you would find in practice. I recall my first practical station was Laboratory Diagnostics and I was so relieved to see a microscope that looked something like the one I had in practice – I thought 'maybe I could pass this exam'!

As I mentioned earlier, OSCEs are not a quiz on your knowledge of different brands on refractometer or X-ray tube heads. You can ask where the things that you need are: on switches, emergency flush, fresh gas flow outlet. All things that will then allow you to move on and demonstrate your clinical skills in the time allowed.

Other students

There are myths that there is a lot of crying and hysteria in the exam room. In all the times I have examined I have seen people looking like they are controlling tears and nerves, that is normal, it is a stressful day. It is incredibly rare that people cry/are sick/have breakdowns. If anyone does feel unwell, sick or too upset to do a task then there are spare examiners to step in and help. They will help the person feeling unwell and make sure there is minimal disruption to everyone else. If you feel unwell during the exam please alert an examiner. Get some water to drink. Take a deep breath.

If you are near anyone who is upset look away, both of you will feel better and focus on your own breathing. Think about the next task you might get or go through a checklist of your plan to focus your mind on your exam. Make sure you use the exam time for your benefit and do not get distracted by anyone else.

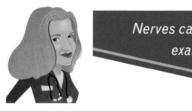

> *Nerves can affect anyone – the examiners can help you.*

Your own nerves

Nerves affect us all. Some people can turn nerves into positive energy (see Chapter One) while others are not that lucky. Be prepared to feel nervous. It means you will cope much better when you are nervous.

It is a myth that some people sail through their exams, they just have a plan in place to cope and it is a good idea to have a plan. This means you focus on yourself, other people are then less likely to distract you and you are thinking of your work, not that of other people.

It is also worth noting that what we remember about the exams is not always reliable. Our brains are not a video camera. Our memories are a compilation of what we have done on the day and previous experiences of the task. This can mean your memory of what you did in a task or station is not exactly what happened. Between stations do not focus on the last task, focus on the next one.

> *'The way to get started is to quit talking and begin doing.'*
> *– Walt Disney*

#OSCEtips #PlanetRVN

Now we have the myths out of the way let us get onto the facts. Every vet nurse will sit a practical exam or OSCE before they qualify. They are an assessment of your clinical skills in an exam situation, confirming your NPL or CSL has been completed and they demonstrate the standards employers would expect of an RVN, Vet Tech or Vet Nurse on Day One of their employment.

You can find access to OSCE tips through the hashtags above – #OSCEtips will provide tips from all medical OSCEs, so some are relevant to vet nursing and some not and #PlanetRVN has my free OSCE videos – some a couple of years old now but still relevant!

Mark sheets – revision aid or not?

An exam where you get the answers! Yay! That's amazing! Just like with MCQ exams surely this means everyone will pass? Well, no. You need to be clinically competent at the task and while the mark sheet may help guide you, your success is a combination of your own work standards, your application of theory and your experience and assessment in work-based learning.

Remember the mark sheets are written for several reasons. Yes, they can help you practise and see how the exam is set up but they are not the only guidance you should have for the exam. Your mentor at work and tutor at college can guide you and do go back to check your theory notes on the subject area.

Exam mark sheets are also written for examiners to use and facilitate structured feedback. That means there are sometimes more steps written than you need as a student. If the task needs you to draw up medication then you are going to put together a needle and syringe in a sterile fashion. You do not need the four or five steps there are on the mark sheet to know that.

> *You don't need to memorise every step of the mark sheet to succeed.*

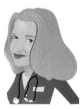

Some people focus on memorizing each step. With around 40 tasks with at least 15 steps each then you are looking at remembering almost 1000 steps, many of which you will do automatically. Even if you are a linear learner and like learning in this way it will probably not help you. There are steps you need to achieve to be safe – for sterility or personal or patient safety, these are areas to focus on, not every single step.

 You can use key steps, or areas that you are worried you might forget, to focus your planning for the exam – but do not get stuck trying to recall every step. It may help to go to the Chapter Five exam prep checklist and use this to help focus your planning so you are not simply working from an exam checklist that was not intended to be a study guide.

Revision for practical assessments

Revision is usually seen as a pen and paper exercise where you sit at a desk and read and write. While you do need to do some reading around the subject and I would suggest writing your own plan for each task, please make sure the majority of your time is spent on more practical and less written revision.

In the stress of an exam your brain wants the security of a familiar path. Therefore, it is better for your exam performance if you have practised each task as thoroughly and often as possible.

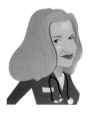

Your brain will go to the most familiar actions in your exam – bad habits will appear!

However much you think you can over-ride your everyday actions they will be where your brain goes to in a stressful situation, which could mean your bad habits from work appear unexpectedly in the stress of an exam.

I would advise you to start your revision by going through your notes and textbooks to find information on how to carry out the skills required in the exam. Check your record of cases nursed, if you have completed one similar as you may have made notes there too. Ask your clinical coach for any information they have.

This can be the starting area for each task: gathering some theory to back up the actions and discussing the exams with your clinical coach. You will probably have already talked about OSCEs with your colleagues throughout your journey but it is good to talk about what to do to prepare specifically for the exams.

Check the subject areas and sort your research into the relevant sections and tasks. Write your own notes of how you demonstrate these skills, as you will already be doing them. Although the exams are set to ensure everyone reaches a set standard of skill level they are still individual in that you can approach completing the task in a way that is comfortable for you. You can then start making a plan for each task as you look at the mark sheet. Try to leave focusing on the mark sheet until after you have started collecting your information. Otherwise it can feel like you have to change what you do to fit the exam and this should not be what an exam is about.

Planning your task

As you get to read the task before you attempt it you can use this time to plan. You have already seen similar task sheets when practising and they do not take long to read, but it can be long enough to start panicking.

To stop the panic, break the task down into manageable sections and plan to attempt those. If calculations worry you then plan to do that first, focus on the equation, the units and use that to stop you worrying.

Making a plan

Writing your exam plan on flash cards can be really useful and allows you to make notes on the tasks and even draw or have a picture of what you want to achieve.

The plan should include the order you may wish to do the task in:

• key steps – safety first!
• calculations

- units
- steps you are worried about – perhaps from previous feedback.

Some tasks have a logical order, while others you can approach in your own way. Some, like anaesthesia, can be carried out in a different way from the way the mark sheet is set out. Remember the mark sheet has many uses and is not intended as your only revision aid.

I have included a possible plan for an anaesthesia task below (Figure 7.1). I split the task into four short sections and there are notes on each area – personalize it to make your own plan – do you need a prompt to remember scavenging or to use the 'in use' label?

I view the task as four mini sections:

1 complete my calculation
2 select and set up circuit

3 carry out machine check
4 carry out circuit check.

This makes it seem achievable and I can focus on one area at a time.

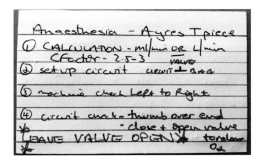 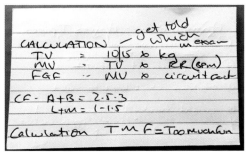

Figure 7.1 Examples of OSCE exam plans (Ayres T piece)

Practising for each task

Each task question gives guidance on how to demonstrate the required skills. The questions are clear and set out what the task involves. But only you know what areas are your strengths and weaknesses. Therefore, exam preparation is always personal to you. While you may find fluid therapy tasks easy, others may struggle with them, and while bandaging is challenging for you, others may find that easy.

Once you have a brief plan for each task, a few lines will do, start to practise it following your plan. Only then will you see if the plan is easy to remember and if it works for you.

Be prepared to go back and revise your plan if it does not feel right. The OSCE exams are a reflection of what you do regularly as a vet nurse, *but* they are exams and so have time limits and often focus on a small part of a larger nursing task. For example, the tube feeding task is usually 6 minutes long, yet we know we would take a lot longer in a ward to achieve this. Our whole task would include reviewing the patient, selecting food, making up the food, if needed, and much more. This is not realistic to examine in a time limited exam, so the focus is on the calculation, safety and administration of a small amount of food. You need to tailor your plan to reflect this so it might feel odd at first doing a select part of your usual routine.

'If you can dream it, you can do it.'
– Walt Disney

Initially practising with a friend is great. It helps you gain confidence and you can discuss what is happening and share your ideas. As you progress you also need to consider how well each practice is going and also how well you critique your work.

Self-assessment

Being able to recognize when something has not gone well and when you need to make improvements is really important. You will know the exams and your strengths and weaknesses better than anyone, so while advice is great and helpful, only you can filter it for your needs.

Assessing yourself is not about being harsh on yourself, it is about being realistic. Starting with the basics – when and where are the best times to practise, and who is the best at advising you?

After a night shift may not be the best time to practise, and trying to identify your instruments during a complicated surgery may not be the best use of your time. It is worth considering when it's best to practise. After hours or on a Sunday afternoon, if you are not in a 24-hour practice may be the better options. Always ask permission to be in the practice outside of normal working hours and share when you are there and when you have left and please try not to be there on your own. This might sound silly but try to avoid lone working if at all possible, especially for opening and closing the building. Make use of the facilities, but be safe.

I know some students have created working groups and met each other at their different practices. This allowed for group practice, safety and gave the opportunity to try different equipment in a safe and supportive environment.

As for who is best at advising you – this is a contentious area! Everyone has slightly different ways to do things. Your clinical coach and college tutor are the best first options to go to with questions. You can also speak to people who have recently passed their exams. You also need to build up a network of people who can support you. While it is great to have a 'cheerleader', always try to have someone who will be truthful about how well you are doing, tactful, but truthful.

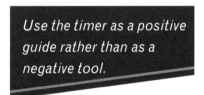

Use the timer as a positive guide rather than as a negative tool.

I would also add here that you need to start timing your practising early on. It is a great way to see how much better you are getting and, unless you time yourself, you will have no idea if you are completing the tasks in the allotted time.

Creating exam conditions

After some time practising it can feel that you have pretty much got this OSCE exam stuff sorted. You have critiqued yourself, you are not going over the time. You have got a plan in your head and you are sticking to it.

What more can you do? Well, there is the added exam stress of the examiner. Probably someone you do not know, who will stand and watch your every move. This can be quite off-putting, even intimidating. There is also the aspect of both physically and mentally moving from one task to another, and managing the time in between where you need to remain calm.

Can you replicate the exam experience before you get there? It will give you an idea of how you will cope with these extra aspects of the exam, like using the time to read the task in the time given and waiting without worrying between stations. You could set up two or three tasks and attempt them sequentially. Perhaps have a person, who you normally do not have contact with, 'examine' you: a vet you do not often work with or a nurse from another practice? This will make it feel more like an exam and if you can have someone time each task, the breaks in between, and the time taken to read each task it will really give you the opportunity to see how you will cope with the exam set up.

Group practising

You may well have friends sitting their exam at the same time as you or you may be allowed to practise in college time. Both are great opportunities to watch others and share information, although keep to the facts and avoid the myths!

I know some people prefer not to practise with others but there are benefits. It can help you get over being shy or having stage fright, and this is helpful for your exam. While I have heard students say they will be fine on the day with the examiner as they are assuming they will not know them but, you never know who your examiner will be. It may be an ex-colleague or tutor so you need to be prepared there could be someone there you know. Practising with people you know can help prepare you for this.

Group practising also lets you watch other people do tasks and this can be a very good way to learn different options of completing tasks. This can be particularly helpful if you do not have this particular piece of equipment in your practice or if you feel you could improve the way you do things.

The feedback you get in a group can feel less intimidating than 1 to 1. When the whole group discusses a problem it can seem more manageable as everyone experiences similar issues. Everyone will have their own coping strategies and you can share your views and learn from others.

Creating exam equipment

As the exams will take place on mannequins there is the issue of learning how to handle a fake patient. This is easily rectified as there are numerous medium to large stuffed toys that can be bought and used.

You will need a long legged soft toy for bandaging and X-ray tasks. Further rigidity for bandaging can be added to fore limbs by placing a wooden baton inside the toys leg, although it is not strictly necessary.

For other tasks, smaller patients are suitable. Students have told me they have found soft toys in charity shops that have worked well. You should consider a soft toy for:

- injection tasks
- tube feeding
- urinary catheter
- ear/leg swabs
- kennel cleaning

- handling and restraint
- bandaging
- X-ray
- fluids.

One patient could be used for more than one task, it is not uncommon to find vet practices with a toy that has an indwelling urinary catheter, a naso-gastric tube and wounds to its legs.

> 'There's nothing funnier than the human animal.'
> – Walt Disney

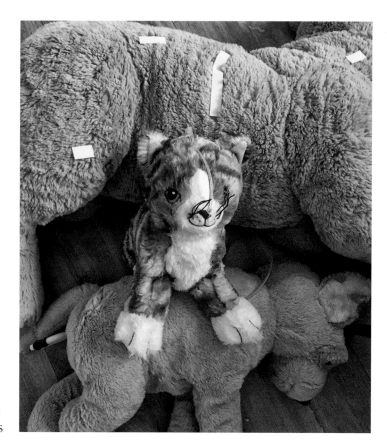

Figure 7.2
Homemade mannequins

Learning information – different approaches

Learning facts and information can seem disconnected from what you do every day with your patients. To help you learn, you can consider a few different approaches after the usual note making. Some of these can really help boost your study morale and make the whole experience seem more positive.

Mnemonics – 'neemonics'

I like to use **mnemonics**. These are where you have a list of information and you take the first letter of each word and make an easy to remember phrase from it, see the flash card in Figure 7.1, 'Too Much Fun' is a way to recall the anaesthesia calculation.

Too	Tidal volume
Much	Minute volume
Fun	Fresh gas flow

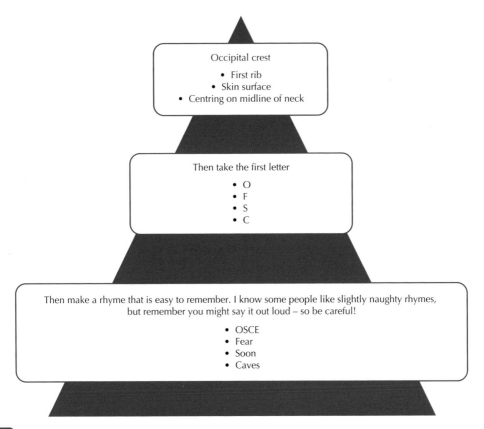

Occipital crest
- First rib
- Skin surface
- Centring on midline of neck

Then take the first letter
- O
- F
- S
- C

Then make a rhyme that is easy to remember. I know some people like slightly naughty rhymes, but remember you might say it out loud – so be careful!
- OSCE
- Fear
- Soon
- Caves

Figure 7.3 Revisiting the Mnemonics creator

In Chapter Four, on MCQ exams, there is some more information on mnemonics and memory techniques, with rhymes, songs and more.

On the day

There is an On the Day guide online. You should also consider what you will be wearing for OSCEs. You are usually required to be in uniform, have hair tied back (if long) and have no false nails or nail varnish. Have you got that planned?

Your uniform does not have to be a stripy traditional student vet nurse version – it can be whatever you wear to work. Just make sure it looks presentable, is clean and most importantly comfortable for you to wear.

In the exam, the examiner expects to see someone who looks professional and acts professionally. As an examiner, I am pleased to see candidates who are smiling and making eye contact with me, even if it is clear they are nervous. It indicates that a student is prepared to do their best and is ready to attempt the task in front of them.

Then on the day you can focus on what you need to do.

Nerves

It is normal to be nervous. People who say they do not get nervous are either lying or they turn nerves into positive energy and do not think they are nervous (see Chapter One for a more in depth look at nerves).

I would always advise to be prepared for nerves and plan to harness the extra energy that adrenaline surge brings.

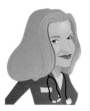

Breathe.
Read the task.
Do the task asked.
Check the task instructions before you leave the station.

In the grand scheme of things this is all you need to do! Yes, I know there is more, but it is a start. Once you have your mind focused on your breathing you need a plan to Do the task asked – check out the Make a plan section above.

Should they be videoed?

I have heard people arguing that there would be no issues with OSCEs results if they were recorded by video. This has been debated in other sectors that use them and research has shown that a large number of cameras would be needed to accurately film all aspects of a practical task, and this would still not be 100% foolproof. The recording would also need to be viewed by examiners to determine if the student had passed or not and so examiner discretion is still relied upon.

It is a shameless plug, but please see www.janervn.com for my videos on YouTube to see what it is like filming OSCE tasks. It is hard enough completing a task in front of an examiner let alone worrying about cameras. I am doing the tasks for the camera and there are some tasks like bandaging that are hard to do when facing a camera.

I hope many of these myths can now be put to bed and let students and clinical coaches together focus on working towards passing these exams with the minimum of stress – it's all that everyone wants!

Different types of assessment

As I mentioned at the start of the chapter there are variations on the OSCE as a practical assessment. These include **OSPVEs**, DOPS and case-based assessments. The assessment goal remains the same, that it is to assess clinical competence, these are just variations. As we progress and wish to examine more complex tasks, including communication skills and professionalism, OSCEs in their current format will not be suitable.

> 'We keep moving forward, opening new doors, and doing new things, because we're curious and curiosity keeps leading us down new paths.'
> – Walt Disney

OSPVEs

Objective Structured Practical Veterinary Exams have been used most commonly at the Royal Veterinary College in the UK. They are used across vet and vet nursing courses and are very similar to OSCEs but are used to assess skills outside the clinical area too.

DOPS

Directly Observed Procedural Skills (DOPS), also referred to as Direct Observation of Procedural Skills are used in the workplace as an assessment of practical skills.

Apart from the setting, which may be in the workplace, as a candidate in the exam you probably will not notice much of a difference between being in a DOPS or an OSCE station. Your preparation might be different as the mark sheet is usually not available prior to the assessment and as it is structured differently, it is not the prescriptive list of steps an OSCE has. While I am sure many students will wail at this as they rely on the OSCE mark sheet, the structure of a DOPS is beneficial to students. The less didactic marking criteria allows for a wider variety of student actions to be declared competent. This flexibility allows for multiple observations with different situations, so the student is not disadvantaged by being assessed either in the workplace or the clinical skills lab.

CEX

The Clinical Evaluation Exercise takes place in the workplace. It is a longer assessment than an OSCE or a DOP and involves assessing communication, patient conduct, taking histories and a clinical exam of a patient. They are rarely used in vet training and at the moment are not used in vet nursing as they increase the cost of assessment in both time and staffing. The existing practical exams are already an expensive form of assessment.

The CEX was replaced by the mini-CEX where a shorter assessment time of around 15 minutes is used. This format has proved as reliable and as it is shorter they can be used more freely and frequently, with some vet programmes running four to six per year. The feedback is given in the form of an action plan to support future learning so these assessments can also be used early in training.

> 'All our dreams can come true, if we have the courage to pursue them.'
> — Walt Disney

There are more assessments of practical skills, however, these are used more in work-based learning and so will be covered in Chapter Eight.

 Review Chapter 7 and how to apply what you have learned with the Reflective Template.

Chapter Seven glossary

Competency Standards – VNCA educational standards (Australia)
Day One Skills – RCVS educational standards
Essential and Recommended Skills – AVMA educational standards (USA)
mnemonics – a memory aid using acronyms
OSCE – objective structured clinical exam, assessment of clinical skills
OSPVE – objective structured practical veterinary exam, OSCE system devised at RVC London
practical exam – similar to OSCE, an assessment of clinical skills

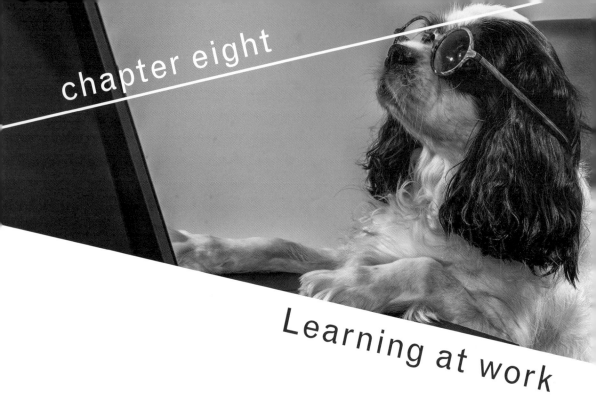

Learning at work

What is learning at work?

Work-based learning (WBL) and assessments are used in many countries as a core part of the vet nurse qualification and can provide a record of the nursing skills carried out and patients nursed. In other countries there is not always a focus on practical skills or WBL. This is one of the reasons that the UK programme is rated so highly, as vet nurses start their career with a wide range of approved skills – through the UK Day One Skills.

Other training schemes that have a practical element include:

- US Vet Techs – Essential and Recommended Skills
- Australian Vet Nurses – Competency Standards
- South African vet nurses.

In the UK we call this type of learning WBL, in Australia it is on the job (**OTJ**) training and in many US states it is referred to as the student taking an **externship** (Ex). This is similar to a

> *For ease of reading I will use WBL as the term for this chapter, rather than put WBL|OTJ|Ex each time!*

UK **internship**, which may be a more familiar term for some people. Whatever it is called it means that part of your training involves working in a real practice with real clients, real patients and professional colleagues.

WBL may be part of the assessment for your course and is carried out by trained staff at work. It is different to college assessments in that it takes place over a longer period of time and is a collaboration between you and your support team. In the UK, the current term for the main person supporting you is a **clinical coach** (CC) but previously they have been called assessors (see Appendix A for more on clinical coaches). For vet nursing schemes in the UK there is one person identified as being your CC but the whole practice is involved – it is a 'training practice'. In other schemes, different titles may be used, during this book I will use the title clinical coach. I was going to use the general title supervisor but as your employment supervisor may be different to your training supervisor I thought that might get a bit confusing.

With this assessment method you are showing evidence of your improving skills throughout your training. You are required to record the cases you have been involved with you are showing where you have gained your experience, across a variety of patients and cases.

Why is it used?

WBL has many benefits. It gives the student access to real-life situations while being supported. This allows a time for students to develop their professional decision making and professional relationship skills. They can add theory to practice and be assessed in the work environment.

Being assessed in different ways is beneficial for students as it shows their abilities in different environments. The feedback received is different in the workplace than the college environment and can be seen as 'real' by some students as it is from colleagues. Magnier and Paed (2017: 266) state: 'One of the great strengths of work-based assessment methods is their ability to document the humanistic aspects of a clinical encounter.'

By humanistic they mean to assess the person's ability to treat others with respect and communicate well and be part of a team. These things are hard to assess in college yet are essential traits in vets and nurses.

'No matter what people tell you, words and ideas can change the world.'
– N.H. Kleinbaum, Dead Poets Society

An issue faced by all vet nurse and vet courses is that there are so many things to assess. We vet nurses graduate with skills and knowledge spread across sciences, arts and communication, as well as research and presentation skills. Making sure every student reaches their competence level is not an easy task. Getting help from colleagues via the clinical coach WBL scheme in the UK and OTJ and other assessments in other countries is needed and very beneficial to all. WBL also allows students to develop their professional decision-making skills with real patients and clients with the support of qualified staff.

Showing your experience

In the UK student vet nurses are required to keep a record of the patients they care for during their training. This is via an online record called (currently) either the nursing progress log (NPL) or clinical skills log (CSL). This will be discussed in this chapter and while not used for every vet nursing student across the world the advice on team working and reflection are beneficial to all. I will use NPL as the 'name' for this record as it is currently the most widely used term in the UK.

The NPL requires a student to have a named CC and for the practice to be registered as a training practice. The training practice designation requires that it is the whole practice that provides training. There is a named point of contact for the student and college, but it is the whole team at the practice that are involved in providing the training.

The NPL is created from a **process** of demonstration, learning, reflection and becoming **competent** in the skills asked. This means a suitable skilled person shows the student the appropriate way to carry out a task, referencing Day One Skills, the college syllabus and assessments (including OSCE tasks), the RCVS vet nurse code of conduct and their own research. The Day One skills and RCVS code of conduct are both available for free online. You can also access the American Veterinary Medical Association (AVMA) and Veterinary Nursing Council of Australia (VNCA) information for comparison – links are in the resources. The college syllabus will be available to the student and to the clinical coach.

While this is the UK system there are parts of the process that can be used in most practical training situations. The whole team needs to be involved in training new staff, including vets and nurses. There should be a named contact for the student to discuss their training and be a point of contact for others involved in the training. This person should be a registered member of the vet or vet nursing team. The clinical coach should have the skills to access information to research the industry standards for clinical skills and be prepared to learn these themselves and be able to share this with others.

The named person, or CC, does not need to be the sole person to demonstrate all the skills across the programme. This is unrealistic as it is a large workload and there are likely to be others who can demonstrate certain skills better. This shares the work load and helps the student to realize the CC is not the only provider of information.

The CC does need to make sure that the people used in training the student are using the correct techniques and information. People other than the CC who take part in the training process are called professional witnesses in the UK. They can demonstrate **tasks**, watch a student's performance and decide if they are competent. Witnesses need to be either a registered vet or vet nurse or have skills and qualifications relevant to that task. Areas where witnesses are commonly used include:

- equine skills
- laboratory skills – where there is a skilled lab technician
- reception and communication skills – receptionists and practice managers
- anaesthesia
- exotic patients
- bandaging.

As many student vet nurses have spent some time in practice before starting official training using the NPL, there may be some tasks they already do well. To reflect this there is an option called 'quick start'. This is where the CC decides there is no need to demonstrate a skill as the student does this task to the standard required already. This means the student can start to log cases and should need fewer cases to become competent. They still need to log cases to cover the potential case differences, such as species or age range, however, once these have been completed the student may well feel competent.

What is competency?

I have used the word 'competent' several times and it is now a good time to explore what this means. To complete tasks and have them signed off as completed the CC has to know the student is competent. The student has to ask for this to happen so both parties need to feel confident that the student is competent in the skill in question.

We all go through a process when learning of moving from the learning stage to competent to proficient to expert. These stages are taken from work by Dreyfus who suggested a five-stage model.

Novice Has an incomplete understanding, approaches tasks mechanistically and needs supervision to complete them.

Advanced beginner Has a working understanding, tends to see actions as a series of steps, can complete simpler tasks without supervision.

Competent Has a good working and background understanding, sees actions, at least partly, in context, able to complete work independently to a standard that is acceptable, though may lack refinement.

Proficient Has a deep understanding, sees actions holistically, can achieve a high standard routinely.

Expert Has an authoritative or deep holistic understanding, deals with routine matters intuitively, able to go beyond existing interpretations, achieves excellence with ease.

Adapted from Dreyfus (2004).

The standard in the UK for Day One Skills for vet nurses is to be competent or above at the prescribed skills. The level of skill achieved across the tasks required for the NPL will vary. Some tasks that are carried out frequently will be done at a level higher than competent, compared to those tasks not under-taken so regularly. It is good for student and CC to remember that the level required is competent – someone who can work independently in the majority of situations that occur in the practice, can ask for assistance in more unusual situations and can help others with their work.

Being competent includes the attributes above and:

- being able to work independently in most circumstances
- carrying out tasks without the need to access help
- recognizing where you might need help
- knowing where to access that help.

Many students aim to achieve proficient to expert before being signed off and this can delay their progress and put too much pressure on them and their CC. Students and CC need to accept that there are some tasks that students will only become proficient to expert in once they have been qualified. This is because they may need exposure to more cases than they would see in their training period or because a skill needs them to be better at other tasks before improving skills in this area. This is particularly true of emergency and critical care cases and nursing for specific disease processes. Moving beyond com-petent is also not equated with doing the tasks specifically quickly or taking short cuts. While the student or CC may feel 'it's nice' to have certain cases logged as experience, the record of cases should reflect the life in practice the student has led.

To stop yourself becoming overly focused on improving the skill level far beyond competence to the detriment of your progress is to ensure you are being realistic about the cases seen and that you are using their reflective comments properly to chart your progress. With this it is time to look at reflection for WBL.

> 'You'll never have that kind of relationship in a world where you're afraid to take the first step because all you see is every negative thing 10 miles down the road.'
> – Sean Maguire, Good Will Hunting

Judgement of your own skills

- Can you complete a task from beginning to end without asking for guidance?
- Can you complete a task in reasonable time?
- Can you complete a task and there is no need to get an experienced member of staff to check it?
- Do you manage some areas of the practice on your own during shifts?
- Do you check textbooks or notes before completing tasks?

Reflection for WBL – the differences

We use reflection a lot in education. Academic assignments in vet nursing courses often ask for reflection on a case previously cared for. This is reflection on action – reflecting after the fact. Reflection for WBL often means you need to reflect *in* action and this can be much harder as you are using reflection for improvements in clinical skills. Head back to Chapter One to revisit reflection.

For reflection on action we usually look at two aspects of our actions:

- What have you learnt?
- What will you do differently next time?

This is pretty simplistic but as an overview of reflection on action it sums up what we do, if you want to go a bit further you can consider expanding your thoughts:

- Create headings to make your notes easy to review.
- Did it relate to your objectives/thoughts at the start of the session or course?

Reflection is usually based around the cycle of – plan, do, record, reflect – this may sound difficult to achieve while we are carrying out a task or action. We do not need to get stuck on the planning at this stage as it will happen as probably the last part of the cycle. We can also make reflection feel more like an activity in the present by considering what reflection asks you to do – it wants you to review your actions and apply what you think about them. This is very personal as your actions are unique to your situation in the practice, in your education and your skills set. Only you can review your activities and decide what to do in the future. Instead of reflection – which sometimes has poor connotations think of review and apply – R&A.

I have found with teaching students R&A that there comes a point where you have to make sure it is a positive experience. The process should not become one where you are negative about yourself, and this includes deciding when to stop with the reflective cycle. This is especially true for clinical skills where you may not get the chance to practise them again immediately. For clinical learning and improvement consider using the following as a way to guide your reflection:

- needs are met – for that individual patient
- needs are met – for your overall body of knowledge/skills. (May, 2017)

You need to be aware of the categories of competent, proficient and expert, and be honest with yourself about which you are trying to achieve. We all want to be the best we can be, but you cannot achieve expert status in all aspects of clinical skills as a student and nor should you want to.

Identifying when your new learning is enough is important – when you are confident you achieve the task in the majority of situations, when you feel you can start and complete the task independently and you are able to support others in doing the task. Yes, you could go and learn more but you need to use your time wisely with so much to achieve.

Reflection, R&A, whatever you want to call it is individual to the person and the practice, and it does not have to be a laborious process. You may wish to check the templates available for download.

Reflective comments and how they work

With the NPL in the UK a reflective comment is required for each case logged. This might sound like a lot of work. However, the comment is meant to be short – a sentence or phrase to get a picture of your feelings and ability about a task that builds up over time. There is little point writing a big comment for the first case, nothing for the next three cases then deciding you are competent on the fifth case. It does not let you or your CC know how you feel, how you have improved and what you have done to achieve being competent, it would suggest you have not considered this yourself.

Reflective comments about your own actions can be very hard to write down and sometimes hard to keep positive. Many people feel reflection is a way to be negative about themselves, and it really is not. It is important that you learn a way to make short, positive comments that review your actions and apply some feedback to take forward to the next attempt.

It is important to stay positively critical of your actions and always have a way to move forward. If an attempt at a task does not go as well as you liked, consider what was not ideal from more than one viewpoint. You have to look at your actions, but also your feelings and the impact of your environment. Reflect on your actions as each of these:

- your role as a vet nursing student
- your personal feelings/situation
- you as part of the veterinary team/practice
- as a prospective vet nurse on the register.

There are many things that will impact on your actions, so ensure you reflect on these things too. It may be easier to reflect on the four roles above separately to begin with so you can understand the differing reactions there are to the actions you did. Do not be afraid to include information on your own health and well-being. If this features a lot then please do write down for yourself your feelings and speak to someone. Vet nurse training is hard, do not make it worse by thinking that every case log has to be like a Famous Five book, *Five Go Vet Nursing*, where it is all positive and jolly and there is lashings of ginger beer.

Write a brief draft of your reflective comment. You could use a template similar to ones we have used before in this book – see Chapters One, Seven and Nine. Using the four viewpoints listed above you could create a table (see Table 8.1) to note your comments, review if you need further help, where you could get it and then summarize this for your reflective comment on your NPL.

Table 8.1 Work-based learning reflection table

Case/skill/situation	Positives	Negatives	Plans for the future
Personal – your personal feelings/ situation			
Professional – SVN student			
Personal and professional – as part of the veterinary team/practice			
Professional – prospective vet nurse on the register			

It may help you to head back to Chapter One and review the work on reflection there, or access the reflective templates available online.

> 'You must strive to find your own voice because the longer you wait to begin, the less likely you are going to find it at all.'
> – N.H. Kleinbaum, Dead Poets Society

Working in a practice

These next few sections focus on the UK training scheme but the following sub-sections still have useful information so do not skip right to the end of the chapter if you are not UK based (see Appendix B for some guidance on student–practice contracts). Some of these areas will be relevant to all students and I'll focus on:

- spotting appropriate cases for your skill level
- managing the workload
- simulating cases
- working with your training support.

Spotting cases – relevant to ALL vet nurse training

Every patient or client you work with is a potential case to improve your skills, learn more and record as evidence of your progress. This sounds great but can be a little overwhelming. Which are the best cases to choose and how many of each should you record and when? Is recording every phone call from a morning on reception the best use of time and has it taught you anything?

It can seem that it is best to pick the 'exciting' and different cases to record as evidence of your progress. While for certain areas the cases are all different, such as in emergency care, in many areas the skills you need to be competent on are the everyday skills. Being able to clean kennels, run lab work and triage patients over the telephone are all skills that are required daily when working as a veterinary nurse.

Choosing cases should be guided by several factors:

- cases coming into the practice
- staff availability
- rota
- scheme of work from university or college
- CC guidance
- personal skill level.

This may sound like a lot of things to consider when looking for cases but much of it is common sense and will naturally occur in the workplace.

This is where working well with your team is essential. I would advise that you take responsibility for finding out as much of the information needed as you can before planning what to achieve with your CC.

To get the best out of your work based placement you need to be aware of:

- your rota – where you are
- your colleagues – who is available to help you
- your skill level
- your scheme of work.

Consider these two scenarios where you could gain experience and log cases.

Scenario A

You are on the rota to work in lab next week. You have several tasks open as you have spent time there before with your CC. On next week's rota, you are there for one day with an RVN and one day on your own.

You want to log as much as possible on the open tasks as you need to increase your number of completed tasks. You also still have some tasks to open.

Plan to open the new tasks on the day with the RVN working with you. Select three tasks that are either commonly done in your lab, or for which you know there are patients in requiring those lab tasks.

Check the consult diary and the in-patients. Consider your college work, both in terms of lab knowledge but also disease processes or anatomy. If you are learning about the urinary system or renal disease or diabetes then urinalysis will feature. Perhaps that could be a focus?

Check with your CC that they agree with your choice of tasks and that they approve of the staff member who will demonstrate them to you, as all witnesses need your CC's approval. You can then ask the RVN if they can work with you on the tasks selected. They might want prior warning to brush up on their skills!

On the day where you are on your own, check who is available to help if you need it and then focus on logging cases for the tasks already open. You cannot ignore the other lab work so make sure patients' needs are the priority.

Scenario B

You are working your first weekend shift and have heard it can be hard to get emergency cases so you are looking forward to seeing if there are more emergency cases on a weekend.

You know there is an RVN and a vet working with you for the entire shift and the consultations are usually fully booked. You have some emergency experience but nothing open on your cases. Therefore, bear in mind that the vet and nurse will need to show you new tasks and you will have to demonstrate back that skill for it to be open. There may not be time to do both parts during a weekend but you can get your CC to log each stage separately so you do not lose any cases.

Emergency cover will always require the important skills of fluid set up, theatre set up, appropriate kennel set up and excellent client care. As your skills in these areas improves you will be of more use in an emergency setting and will move on and expand your skills further.

Also consider where you are for college. If you have recently looked at nursing care plans perhaps that is an area to focus on, particularly in emergency medicine care plans, where regular reviews will feature heavily.

Every case is important, logged or not. Making sure the patient is safe and you improve your skills safely is more important than using every case you see for recording purposes.

I am afraid I need to mention the 'R' word here already. Part of the process of WBL is reflecting on your experience. Remember our reflective questions earlier in the chapter? They can help us here, but for now consider planning using the four-point plan from above.

- Where am I in the practice?
- Who am I with?
- What am I able to do and what is new?
- What have I learnt recently from college?

These questions will help you target the best cases for you at the best time. You may be learning about anaesthesia at college but are in wards for the next week. That does not mean you do not use the cases you are working with. You need to look at what you already have open and so can log, or what you feel ready to open when a patient with that need comes in. If you have been focused on studying anaesthesia at home you may wish to check the tasks on the NPL and make yourself a list of what you feel able to try and have the list ready to discuss with your CC when you are next on the rota in theatre. This then helps you stop thinking about the anaesthesia tasks you could be doing and makes you focus on the area you are in.

'There's a time for daring and there's a time for caution, and a wise man understands which is called for.'
– N.H. Kleinbaum, Dead Poets Society

Focusing on the appropriate skills area at the right time involves reflection – especially when considering what you feel comfortable doing on your own, what you need help with and what is totally new. Don't forget that!

Managing the workload

Training as a veterinary nurse is always much harder work than you think it will be. I can say that from personal experience and from the feedback I get from students. The course requires a number of sacrifices and time is the first one. It does not matter which route you study through, there is little spare time. The WBL aspect can seem the hardest part as not all of it is carried out at work. While your practice may be kind and allow you to access your record of training at work they are not required to allow this during your working day. If you are studying, carrying out online learning and researching for assignments, how are you expected to also record your cases from work?

Although it may feel that you cannot plan for the cases that may or may not arrive in your practice, you can. With the NPL there are unlikely to be many times that a case you see is not relevant to you. Even in the last stages where you are trying to find only a few specific case types you can still find cases every week.

To break down what you need to achieve weekly have a look at the potential planner in the box.

Break the NPL workload down into daily achievements – this allows for better time management for both student and CC.

- Log 3 experiences daily for 5 days per week:

  - Which equals 60 experiences a month (or 75 in a 5-week month)
  - Which equals 600 experiences a year over 40 weeks.

- Plan these experiences to match your rota.
- Increase use of witnesses to spread range of tasks that can be declared competent.
- Organize a timetable for internet access at work outside of working hours.

This will allow a number of experiences per skill as some tasks will need more and some less, with this rate of logging you will remain on track for successful WBL completion within the time frame given. You will most likely need to log a few more cases per week, but this should be the minimum you are aiming for. This is likely to take you 15–30 minutes per day, still with 2 days off a week – or 2 extra days to log if you need more cases.

You will have regular meetings with your CC and a college **tutor** to review your progress. This is not to scare you into doing work but because the course is very intense and it is very easy to slip with one or more aspects of the course and thus slow your time to achievement so their monitoring of your progress is important.

If you are not meeting your targets with your CC or your college it is an idea to check if you are doing or experiencing any of the following:

- not spotting appropriate cases
- over logging for each task
- unsure about declaring competency – claiming too late or too early
- under logging, especially due to being in a busy practice 'I'll see that again next week'
- not committing enough time to collecting cases and logging
- pressure from other deadlines
- practice 'too busy'
- CC is slow to open skills or review your competency
- deadlines passed for logging and claiming
- limited internet access.

It is also an idea to see if your worries about completing the WBL aspect of your course fall into any of the following categories:

- poor time management
- poor judgement of own skills
- lack of time committed to NPL
- lack of time with CC
- access to internet.

This is another area where you need to be honest with yourself. A CC can help you plan your work, can set up witnesses and help identify cases, but they cannot nurse them for you and they cannot log them for you. They cannot know how you feel and how you think you can improve. You are a team in

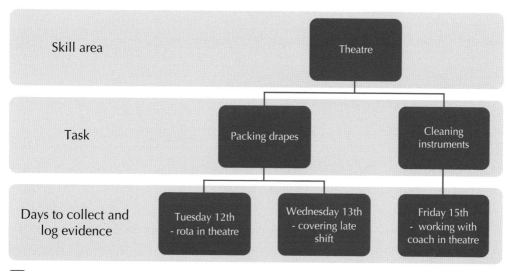

Skill area		Theatre	
Task	Packing drapes		Cleaning instruments
Days to collect and log evidence	Tuesday 12th - rota in theatre	Wednesday 13th - covering late shift	Friday 15th - working with coach in theatre

Figure 8.1 Logging timetable template

achieving the completion of WBL, but the CC needs you to be an independent learner who can think for yourself and ask for the support you need.

Using professional witnesses

As mentioned earlier in the chapter, while there is a single person named as a CC in current training in the UK many people contribute to the training process. Any vet who is MRCVS registered, any RVN or person appointed by your CC can watch your progress and decide if you are competent in a specific area. If not an MRCVS or RVN the person appointed by your CC needs to have significant experience and skill in the given area. For current vet nurse training these areas are usually:

- lab work
- reception
- equine/exotics skills
- imaging.

As these are areas where people with skills, who are not a MRCVS or RVN, are employed for their specific skills, it is always worth checking with the awarding body for your course if these people are required to have area specific qualifi-cations, as proof of these may be required for your records.

Simulations for rarely occurring cases

The recording of skills in the UK is matched to the RCVS Day One Skills. This is a broad range of skills that an RVN is expected to be able to carry out com-petently on their first day as an RVN. Naturally some skills will be used more than others in a practice as they are all different. Where there is a skill that you do not see very often you still need to be competent in it. Remember that competency does not mean being expert or proficient. Owing to the nature of veterinary work most students are expert to proficient in many aspects of their work by the time they qualify. You will most likely have given more subcuta-neous injections than you have taken an elbow X-ray. That's perfectly normal and so do not expect to be as fast or efficient at elbow X-rays as you are at subcutaneous injections.

Working with your CC/supervisor

Your CC may be a vet or a vet nurse (MRCVS or RVN). Both will have had training to be a CC and the support of the practice. However, there will be areas where they will need other people to help. As a student, you need to be aware of and respond to the needs of the practice and the CC. Be prepared to learn from all members of the team. Everyone with experience in the veteri-nary field has something to teach you, from care assistants and reception staff to the practice principal.

As I mentioned before, you will get the most from WBL by being an inde-pendent learner. This does not mean that you work in isolation, it means you have the ability and confidence to recognize your strengths and weaknesses and ask for help with them. This might sound like not being a student! Surely if you knew your strengths and weaknesses you would sail through and not need any help at all. Well, no. You are still learning new things, and also learning about yourself. Being too reliant on a tutor or CC can hold you back as they cannot sit the exams or nurse your patients.

To help you get the best from the coaching and mentoring process it can help to know how that process works. The next section is an extract from some course work for a coaching and mentoring certificate I completed and is an introduction to the coaching process, it shows the relationships needed for successful coaching and some of the models and processes commonly used – in particular **SWOT**, **GROW** and SMART.

Coaching models – what both parties need to know

The workplace coach is in a relationship with the **coachee**. To make this relationship work the coach should display certain characteristics. They should be organized with regard to their approach and commitment to

> *The coach needs to have the affirmation of the organization to show that coaching is a legitimate behaviour or characteristic.*

the coaching task, ensuring there is time to see their coachees and time for work or tasks to be assessed within the agreed time frame. This shows the coach has a commitment to the process. The coach should also be consistent in their approach, ensuring the coachee is not left confused or unsure of the next step in the process. The feedback provided should be participative and objective, both key characteristics that show the process of feedback is meaningful and relevant and easier for the coachee to apply to their situation. The ideal coach should be knowledgeable in the area they are coaching. They need to strike a balance between being tough and authoritative and flexible enough to be balanced and fair. Overall, they should be realistic about the process and be confident enough to stop a process that is not working and make changes to improve the changes and to ensure success.

Use of contracts in training and coaching

Managing the relationship between coach and coachee is very important. Setting out a contract that includes the goals and suggested pathways to achieve the goals is important to securing a positive initial response to the process from the coachee at the prospect of being coached. Therefore, a contract should be agreed upon as part of the initial stages of coaching. You should be able to agree your goals, who you discuss this process with, bearing in mind confidentiality of both parties and also the employer. This contract should be written in a way that allows it to be used as a reference point to check the progress of the coaching process. Including a suggested timeline for task completion allows the contract to make SMART targets. These can be used for feedback and to show if progress is being achieved to the agreed time scale.

Thus, in the contract or in future support sessions the goals for training are agreed between you both, and the targets set match the SMART criteria. This is a good thing to bear in mind while you train. Yes, you have your work based part of your course to consider and it must be completed by the end of your course – but think of it in small, manageable chunks. As before, work

SMART targets

- S – specific
- M – measured
- A – achievable/agreed upon
- R – realistic
- T – timely

that around your rota and the staff available. There is little point stressing about getting the emergency section of your assessment done if you are on the rota for dispensary duties for the next few days. Focus on that instead.

Your CC may well use a coaching model. It allows the coaching process to be set out for the coachee to see and agree to, and it can be used to chart progress. Using a coaching model such as the GROW model (see Figure 8.2) at the start of the process is beneficial as it charts:

- G – Goals – the goals to be set
- R – Reality – the current reality of the coachees' position
- O – Options – the options available in the reality to achieve the goals
- W – Way forward – the way forward using the information gathered answering the points above.

It can be beneficial to have the coach and coachee fill out a GROW model independently. This will show both parties where their personal realities are and it can then trigger some important questions of the GROW coaching process. Open questions should be used initially to get as much information as possible. Setting long-term goals provide the standard that you agree to

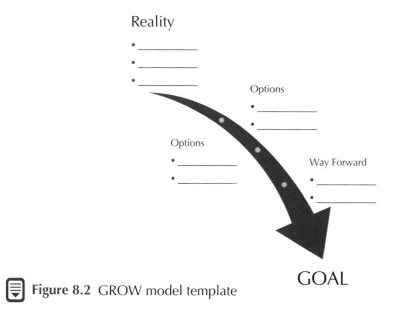

Reality

Options

Options

Way Forward

GOAL

Figure 8.2 GROW model template

work to. The questions can then break down the goals needed to achieve the long-term goal and set a timeline for achievement. Any barriers, perceived or actual, can also be identified and plans set in place to remove them. The use of a coaching model can be as simple or as advanced as you make it. Even with a simple version of GROW, reviewing it regularly at planned times will add new layers as the coach and coachee discover more about themselves and the goals they have set. Reviewing the GROW process allows the initial plan to be adhered to and stops the coaching process being taken off track by other events. However, as mentioned previously, the coach should be strong enough to use the GROW model to see if the process is working and stop or alter it as required.

Similar to the GROW model is the SWOT model of coaching (see Figure 8.3). This can be used by you or your CC and I think it can be used well alongside your NPL or other case based system as it highlights looking for 'opportunities' such as suitable cases.

- S – strengths
- W – weaknesses
- O – opportunities
- T – threats.

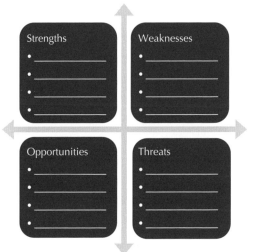

 Figure 8.3 A sample SWOT model

Other tools to assess learning that can be beneficial to WBL include the use of some diagnostic tools that can support the coaching process. These include tools that look at academic ability, learning styles and leadership styles, as discussed in Chapter One. All contribute to allowing the coachee to own their learning and coaching by providing information regarding their skills and abilities.

Tools that you and your CC can use to help find out more about your skills, learning styles and motivation include the following.

- BKSB for academic ability in English and maths.
- The coach can also ask for a skills match, which would show which areas the coachee has similar skills to the skills required and where extra teaching may be required.
- Learning styles questionnaires such as VAK (see Chapter One) or Honey and Mumford can also be used. These can show the coachee how best they can cope with learning new things and how best to prepare for that learning process, that is, whether they are a visual learner or an activist.
- Questionnaires on leadership styles can also help show the coachee the advantages and disadvantages of the way they react to managing others, and how to focus on the positives of *their existing skills set.*

The coaching and mentoring role can be carried out in many different ways but the measure of success will always be your progress, working well together is key to that so it is worthwhile as a student understanding what your coach or mentor is trying to achieve.

Feedback

One of the areas that can be difficult in the workplace is getting and giving feedback, yet it is the basis of all our education. It can be especially hard to receive feedback in the workplace as it can be given:

- by a friend/long-term colleague
- verbally, giving you little time for reflection, unlike written feedback
- immediately, close to the event happening when things are still 'raw', in contrast to academic feedback received maybe days or weeks later when things have settled down.

When receiving feedback, it can be hard to differentiate between your skills and you as a person. Those giving the feedback can fail to differentiate, and even if they do, you may not interpret it as it was intended, so it can feel a little too personal.

Because of all this it can feel a little overwhelming and can be hard to take in the way it is intended – to improve your skills.

To get the most from feedback you need to consider where you are as a learner and communicate this to your CC. Although they will have established their own idea of where you are, your own personal feelings about certain skills and tasks will play a large part in how you receive feedback and are able to use it to improve.

Understanding feedback

Feedback needs to address what could be improved upon, and also praise and promote the areas you did well in. We sometimes focus on the negative a little too much so always keep in mind that there are two sides to feedback and keep a balanced view of how you are progressing.

You will not progress at the same rate in every aspect of your training so do not be upset or surprised if it takes longer to improve skills in some areas. This will also depend on the cases you see and how often you see them, so it is not all down to your own skills.

Types of feedback

You will find that most feedback can be split into four categories that cover the areas of:

- the task carried out
- the context/process in which the task took place
- personal aspects covering your role as an SVN
- personal aspects individual to you.

If you consider feedback in these categories, or as filters through which to view feedback, then you can start to separate out your emotional response. If you receive feedback that upsets you then it is worthwhile checking if the feedback was about you personally or about the other aspects, of the task, what happened around the task and your role as an SVN. It might be worth checking out the earlier sections on dividing reflection into personal and professional areas to help you, as this can help you make feedback work to benefit you.

Feedback provider

The people who give you feedback are also important and can show how well the team works together. I always have to remind clinical coaches that it is a *training practice* and the practice principal has signed an agreement to provide certain aspects of the student vet nurses' training – which involved the whole team.

However, feedback should aim to be delivered by the person who oversees your training and with whom you have established a relationship. You are more likely to act on working to improve your skills if you have a respectful relationship with the person who gives you feedback. The feedback also works well if the person can give you feedback covering the four aspects above and is able to frame the feedback so it is beneficial to you as the student, to colleagues, the patient and to the nursing profession as a whole – putting what happened into the context of future nursing experiences can be very helpful.

To get the most from feedback received, you need to consider:

- context – where you are now
- behaviour – how your behaviour affects your progress
- impact – the potential impact of your actions
- next step – what can you do to improve?

Working in professional teams

As we can see from this section alone, choosing the right person for the right job is key to getting a professional team to work together. The team structure also needs to reflect the training needs and provide support for those in training and those training them.

There also needs to be a clear team process where the goals of the team are known to all, there is trust between members of staff and good communication.

To create a good student experience you need to be able to work with the team in your clinic.

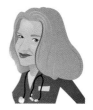

The training process can be mutually beneficial but as the student you do need to make sure you are aware of how the process works and how to make the best of it for your needs.

Having supported a number of students in practice, I have learned that I can never guess how best different people will learn in the workplace – everyone needs to find their own way, with a little support. The more you understand about the types of coaching models and ways of helping you your coach will use, the better you can use them. While you will be using SMART targets to identify how to progress you may find them easier to use as part of the GROW model – I personally prefer the wording of the GROW model and feel it is a more positive way to discuss the boundaries we have in our training. Discussing the *reality* of training in practice always seems nicer than considering the *threats* to progress there may be.

WBL is key to the success of the UK system of vet nurse training – the benefits can also be seen in the US vet tech programmes, the South African programmes and those in Australia and New Zealand.

Learning as part of a supportive team on real cases with real clients is the best learning experience when supported by 'classroom' teaching to supply the theory. I put classroom in inverted commas as there are geographical limitations with traditional classrooms and with improvements in online learning I hope to see an expansion of the provision of courses that offer some traditional face-to-face teaching but allow flexibility with online learning for those not close enough to attend college regularly or able to finance other options of learning.

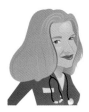
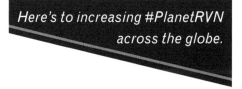

Here's to increasing #PlanetRVN across the globe.

Hidden curriculum

The concept of the hidden curriculum might be new to some readers so I will describe what this means and why it is important to consider it, especially in WBL.

The hidden curriculum is noted in many fields and is particularly present where there is learning in the workplace. It is the concept that there is information taught and learned that is not written in the curriculum or syllabus of a course, yet all students seem to be familiar with it.

In the veterinary world, I think some of these themes that get picked up by vet nursing students include:

- failing OSCEs due to not wearing green
- degree nurses are not as practically capable as diploma nurses
- having a vet as a CC is not as good as having a nurse
- lost practice equipment will not be found by a 'vet look'.

These are not taught aspects of the course but appear as 'myths' about the course and vet world and get repeated with ever increasing emphasis until they seem like the truth. They can have a positive and a negative impact. The ones listed above are more negative, are not true but are still prevalent in the veterinary world.

Where do people get these ideas? They are not taught as part of a syllabus but they can affect the way you work and might change your view of people or patients. They are most often created through informal discussions, and the reactions and body language of your peers and colleagues. These can carry strong messages about the veterinary world that can really make an impression, especially on people new to the industry. Older or more experienced colleagues are very helpful in the training process but their ability to help students with all the obvious parts of the course also means that their own feelings about all aspects of the veterinary world become part of the training.

I have worked with nurses who held strong preconceptions about certain clients or the way certain vets worked that were neither that accurate or helpful. It can be hard to try to work out what will help you and what will not!

The hidden curriculum exists so be aware that all that you learn in your workplace is not always needed or welcome. Part of the process of becoming a vet nurse is learning how to filter information and work on the facts given. This is not easy in such an emotional role but it benefits you and your patients if you can do so.

Work with what you know rather than what you assume.

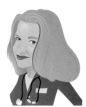

What are the different types of WBL assessment?

In the UK, there are two different ways of recording student vet nurse prog-ress, via the NPL or the CSL. These are online records as per the description at the start of this chapter. While these logs are a record of actual cases that the student has nursed, there is space in WBL for case-based discussion or 'chart exams' based on a simulated case. These could take place in the workplace and could include simulations with mannequins as well as verbal descriptions of decisions made and actions taken.

These types of assessment then start to overlap with the practical assessment discussed in Chapter Seven where OSCE, DOPS and CEX exams are described as ways of testing clinical skills both at college and at work. Heading to the end of Chapter Seven will give you an overview of the differences between these types of assessment.

Case based discussions and 'chart exams' are also very useful for assess-ing communication skills and other skills that aid clinical skills such as team working.

Case-based discussions

These are a formal discussion that is recorded in detail via the assessor. A case that the student has nursed would be chosen in advance and the discussion would provide information about the experience and would allow the asses-sor to ask about additional learning that was carried out and assess the extent of the student's knowledge and decision-making skills.

Previously in the UK, students and CC had professional discussions that were similar to this but where the scenario was a simulation and it provided an opportunity for the student to show knowledge about a certain area.

Chart exams

These are used in human medicine but may become part of the veterinary world as they are a crossover between an OSCE and a communication exam. They allow for some information to be given via a hospital sheet (they are used a lot in the USA and they refer to 'charts' hence the name) and the nurse or doctor then has to work with the patient and carry out the required tasks for their situation.

> *'Carpe diem. Seize the day boys. Make your lives extraordinary.'*
> – *N.H. Kleinbaum,* Dead Poets Society

You could use this style of assessment as a way to simulate situations in practice if you have not seen a particular case for some time to keep skills fresh or to open a new skill. Chart exams are also a great way of simulating emergencies and anaesthesia cases where there is a lot of information to access to set up the case. You can also practice with readings from ECGs, capnographs and pulse oximeters even if you have not got these in practice as there are many online resources from pictures to videos that show the readings from different conditions.

WBL is varied and wide reaching. Different people, places and practices all contribute to an amazing learning experience, if you know how to make the most of it.

 Review Chapter 8 and how to apply what you have learned with the Reflective Template.

Chapter Eight glossary

clinical coach (also mentor/supervisor/assessor) – person taking responsibility for your WBL training and progress

coachee – the student or person who is being coached

coaching – the process of providing support to a student/coachee

competent – a level of skill, deemed the safe level to work on your own and build your skills

externship – scheme to access WBL in America

GROW – goals, realities, options, will

internship – similar to externship, student is assigned to a workplace but may not be an employee

OTJ – on the job training, term for WBL in Australia

placement – student is assigned to a workplace, but may not be an employee

process – how the coaching happens

SWOT – strengths, weaknesses, opportunities, threats

tasks/experiences – terms used for cases you have cared for in the NPL/CSL

tutor – college-based person responsible for teaching/overseeing training

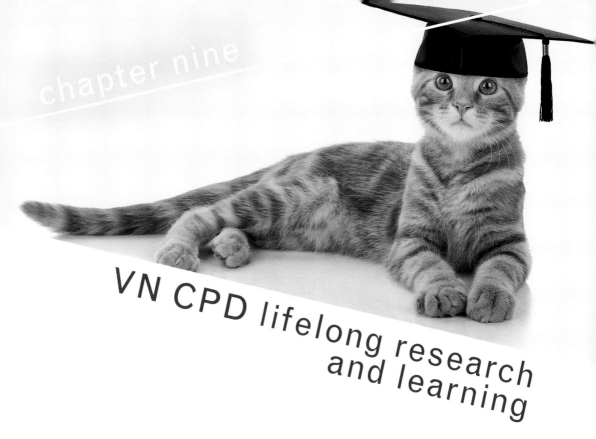

VN CPD lifelong research and learning

Welcome to the end of my book! If you have made it this far – well done. If you have made it this far and implemented any improvements to your studying, then I am really happy and if you are even thinking about making changes and trying new things then I am just as happy.

Chapter Nine is meant for those who are now qualified, a lot of this book is relevant to those studying post-qualification but I thought there are areas of work that we do post-**qualification** that we can all need help with. As vet nurses we are often the key to finding helpful information for the vet and the practice. We get asked to write standard operating procedures (SOPs) and create training protocols for staff.

Where can we get the most up to date and most reliable information to help ourselves, our team and our patients?

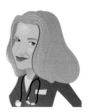

It is also a good time to say that as a vet nurse you will never have all the answers to every situation you find yourself in – and that is absolutely fine! It is the same for vets and other medical professions. However, our reactions to not knowing something can be what stops us learning more. We have levels of knowledge while learning, remember Straus et al. (2010) from earlier in the book.

- That we do know and can recall cognitive resonance.
- That we know we should know but don't/can't recall cognitive dissonance.
- The gaps where we didn't know there was something to know.

Gaps are often created by depth of learning and the need to connect levels of learning, for example, pancreas function learned by rote and applying that knowledge to the disease process of diabetes in cats. These are overlapping knowledge areas but

> 'It is the unknown we fear when we look upon death and darkness, nothing more.'
> – J.K. Rowling, Harry Potter and the Half-Blood Prince

often learned at different times and in different ways, and this can create gaps. Gaps in knowledge are not as scary as you think and are perfectly normal – it is what you do about them that counts.

If you cannot remember something then you need to work on recall so head to Chapters Four, Five and Seven for memory techniques or consider a note book or some other aid to help you remember. You will also find some templates to help you make memory aides for you on the website for this book. You are not expected to be a walking encyclopaedia, but you are expected to know where to get knowledge from when needed. I can never recall nutritional calculations so I have them in my phone so I can check them if needed or can email the file to whoever I am working with – it is good to share.

If you have a gap in your knowledge then you can work towards making that gap smaller. What you need to know will depend on your skills and knowledge and where you work so do not feel you need to know the same as everyone else.

You will be glad to hear that time spent doing research and writing is part of your **continuing professional development** (CPD) requirements if you are regulated. In the UK, the RCVS require vet nurses to do an average of 15 hours CPD

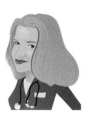

In this chapter, there are a few tips on how to research to find out what you don't know.

each year, or 45 hours over 3 years. There is currently no regulation of CPD providers unless the course has an academic standing, such as a postgraduate course offered by or through a university. However, there are discussions happening around CPD recording at the moment and the idea of an attendees review/rating system on CPD courses has been suggested.

In the USA, the system varies for each state but it is very similar. For example, in California a vet tech needs to carry out 20 hours over 2 years of continuing education (CE). Some CE courses are **RACE** approved. This is a system where the American Association of Veterinary State Boards (AAVSB) have Registry Approved CE (RACE). South African vet nurses are required to gain structured and unstructured CPD points to maintain their listing.

While some CPD may be directed by your role and your employer there is usually a little space for your own choices, so you can make CPD something interesting and individual for you. You could spend time researching and writing on things that interest you, you could think of a question that you feel has not been answered for you, and use your research skills to find the answer.

I will also take a little look at training others, as it can be a key role for many qualified vet nurses. Working out how best to achieve this and still enjoy your role involves reflection, which is a skill you can use in many areas.

'Books are like mirrors: if a fool looks in, you cannot expect a genius to look out.'
– J.K. Rowling, speaking on NBC's Today Show on 20 October 2000

Writing is an important skill, whether it is for your own use, for your employer or for publication. You can become more confident in your writing and editing skills through practice and there are many ways to do this. I will look at the differences and how to write for different needs.

Personal research and CPD

We have covered research in Chapter Two and this is a great start for the usual academic needs of a vet nursing course, and the material there will also help you if you study post-qualification. However, once qualified you may need to research for projects that are individual to you and your practice. The core skills from Chapter Two will help here but you may need to alter a few things to make those skills work for your new needs.

For personal research and CPD you should be focusing on your skills to critically evaluate the resources you find. Once you have left your vet nurse education you may find that access to academic resources is limited. The 'go to' library database you have used may only be available through the university or by paying for access or paying for individual papers.

As described in Chapter Two there are great free or low-cost databases available to you. RCVS Knowledge is around £50 per year for vet nurses and gives access to a huge amount of veterinary research and also *The Veterinary Nurse Journal* and the *Veterinary Nursing Journal* from the BVNA, as well as international journals.

If you are struggling to get access to these then free options include:

- Science Direct
- Google
- Cochrane

- CABAbstracts
- Pubmed.

At this point it is worth highlighting the Cochrane database as it holds an amazing collection of secondary resources (Chapter Two) and provides comprehensive literature reviews of many subject areas. For post-qualification research Cochrane can be a good starting point.

Doctor Google for professional research?

Yes, you can use Google but there are ways to make Google work for you and get it to find the academic research that you want. Google Scholar has had a number of changes to it and while it is still useful, using alternative ways to search the standard Google page can yield better results.

The limitations of Google Scholar include the quality of the research it lists, the variability in available content for all possible areas of research and its ability to show you the most recent research. Google publish what they class as 'scholarly' work but it may not be peer reviewed so the search may include work not suitable for use as references.

By using the standard Google search engine, you search the whole of Google and remove some of these limitations. If you wanted a wide initial search, then it is best to use OR. This would mean you search for 'diabetes cat OR dog'. Then information about either species would show.

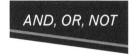

If you use AND between words it looks for data with both these words in. Therefore, searching for information on pet diabetes you could look for 'diabetes cat AND dog' to include both. This will narrow your potential results as any articles that only focus on one species will not show on your search.

Finally, using NOT limits your search in a different way. If you had looked at both searches above and found there was significantly more written about feline diabetes than canine then searching for 'diabetes cat NOT dog' would remove all canine based resources.

Once you have established in more detail what you are searching for it is worth considering how much more detailed your questions could be. If you are searching for information on older cats and diabetes you are starting to add in several key words or phrases into your search. If you put in every possible variable it will take longer and it may not yield exactly what you are looking for.

Head over to Chapter Two to see how to use **Boolean searches** to make Google become more than just a way to find the number for pizza delivery.

Go to an *actual* library

Do not forget that there are local, college and veterinary specific and nursing specific libraries available for you. While there is a huge move towards all research being available online, there are many positives for visiting a library.

Librarians are skilled professionals whose job is to help you find what you need. You should do a little homework before you go to see what the library holds but even many local authority libraries in the UK use Access to Research which is a free to use online search for academic journals.

Many university and scientific publishers are offering articles and journals for free if you visit library branches that participate. If your

Accesstoresearch.org.uk

online database skills are weak then head to Chapter Two and then go to a local library and see what you can find.

Local colleges and some university libraries may be open on day passes for members of the local community. This is most likely at their quieter times, so consider school holidays and see if somewhere close to you has a scheme you can join.

Other libraries

The RCVS has a library at its offices in London. It's free for RVNs on the register to use and while it is easier if you can plan in advance, they are very accommodating if you just pop in. For searches that may include journal articles it is best to book ahead of time and give them an idea of what you need – this saves you time and they can search their stock for you in advance and may find something you did not know was there.

Local college

As with universities local colleges often offer membership to those in the local areas. Many of these types of further education colleges may run animal care or vet nursing courses so you may be surprised at the depth of the information they hold. It is well worth planning what you want to look for and approaching a local college with your planned subject areas.

Vet schools

While the RCVS and some other places I mention are in London, there are vet schools across the world. Again, they often have access to non-students but they will also be keen to support members of the veterinary community.

British Library

I know this is London again, but, it is amazing. A personal favourite of mine. If a building could inspire you then this one will. It's right beside Kings Cross/ St Pancras train stations so easily accessible if you are not in London.

As their collection is so huge much of it is held off site and you do need to order in advance, but they have a 48-hour turnaround and so resources can still be available at short notice. The online database is very easy to use and you can search for specific items or you can search for work in subject areas.

The library has a great online catalogue too and some of the journal articles are available online outside of the library but some you need to visit the library to view them, but with e-copies you do not need to book in advance.

The British Library have great facilities including desks with power points for laptops and great lighting. It is a good place to work even if you do not need access to the information they hold and worth the trip.

In fact, once I have finished this book I am going to take a special trip to the British Library to say an emotional goodbye to this chapter (pun intended) of my life.

Nursing specific libraries

The Royal College of Nursing (RCN) in the UK has nursing specific libraries in Wales, Ireland, England and Scotland. While we have an increasing amount of vet nursing specific research there are still times when we need to look to human nursing evidence. The RCN also has online access that is free for members of the public, so head to their 'search collections' page.

Library collections are added to all the time and new free online access resources are always being developed. Once you have secured your research skills you can use them to assess databases and a wealth of information.

'When in doubt go to the library.' – *J.K. Rowling*, Harry Potter and the Chamber of Secrets

Standard operating procedures

SOPs are among the most common pieces of work vet nurses produce, whether for a practice inspection or to train new staff. An SOP is a way of the practices setting out their individual ways of achieving the common tasks of the vet practice, from how to answer the phone to setting up a temporary isolation unit in a suspected parvo virus outbreak.

There are various templates online to help you start an SOP but they can be as individual as your practice and your team, and should be a reflection of the skills and equipment available to you. You may need to research a huge variety of topics regularly to keep these up to date and you will want to feel confident that the time has been well spent and you have the latest research or product information.

SOPs may mean you need to search academic research as well as government policies and legislation. This can be confusing and time consuming. The important thing to remember is that an SOP is usually a short document and does not need the full Harvard referencing required in assignments for college, which I hope is a little bit of a relief for you. While you do need to keep a record of where the information you found has come from, this can be in your own style as long as it is understandable by other people for future reference.

What are SOPs and how do you start creating one?

An SOP is a system for achieving various tasks that is written down and can be easily followed. They can be used for tasks that are carried out less frequently so you may not recall what to do easily – this might be working out the nutritional needs for a patient with a feeding tube or how to set the answer phone for Christmas opening hours.

Or they may be used for training or standardizing the way certain skills are carried out. If you wish to extend their use they can be used as part of your record keeping and auditing paperwork too.

That's quite a lot to consider so you might want to find out more about writing them.

SOPs are among the most common pieces of research that vet nurses produce, whether for a practice inspection or training new staff.

Templates and flow charts – getting the right structure

There are various templates online to help you start these but they can be as individual as your practice and your team as this should be a reflection of the skills and equipment available to you. The BSAVA have some great guidance on SOPs (see Figure 9.1). You can use Word documents with tables or flow charts, or Excel spreadsheets, both of which are easily printable.

Because an SOP is only ever as good as the thought put into it, it is a great opportunity to check if your protocols are up to date and review them. You might also review who at the practice has been trained in this area and whether any CPD needed.

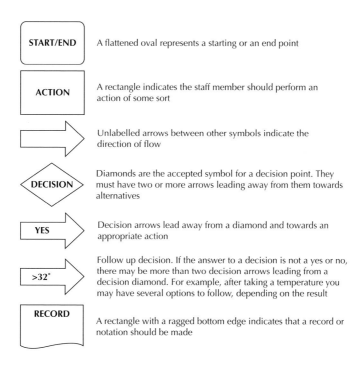

Figure 9.1 Examples of flow charts for tasks reproduced with permission from F. Nind and P. Mosedale, editors. *BSAVA Guide to the Use of Veterinary Medicines.* © BSAVA 2018)

Keeping track of your research

You will need to keep track of the information you find and use, and also any information you choose not to use. This will provide the evidence base for your practices SOPs. It is a good idea to show your evidence to your team and decide together on why and how you carry out certain tasks.

For referencing the information you find, copying and pasting the URL to a Word document is an easy option – but always include the title of the web page and subject area and do keep the date it was accessed. Things move on the web, and you need to make sure even if that URL no longer links you directly to the material, then with the web page title and subject area you can easily search again. For many SOPs, the standard nursing textbooks are also worth checking and City and Guilds have a reading list for the Level 3 Diploma that can help.

The resources you use will be dependent on what topics you are searching and what you want to do. For clinical work, you may need to use the most recent information and you need to be able to assess how good the data is too. Check Chapters One and Two for some digital literacy information.

> *'You need preparing. You need arming. But most of all, you need to practice constant, never-ceasing vigilance.'*
> *– J.K. Rowling*, Harry Potter and the Goblet of Fire

Reflection

> *'Fear of a name increases fear of the thing itself.'*
> *– J.K. Rowling*, Harry Potter and the Philosopher's Stone

This is an area we all probably need to revisit at some point. It is now a key part of vet and SVN training, but for those of us who trained a few years ago it may be something we are less used to.

We use reflection daily without realising it. The start of the reflective cycle is those thoughts about events and situations where you consider that things could have gone better. The basics of the reflective cycle are given in Chapter One, and include a discussion of Teekman, so re-visit that if you need a more in depth reminder. There are reflective templates to download associated with Chapters One and Eight.

As RVNs we also need to consider that CPD may require outcome-based recording. For human nurses in the UK their CPD requires writing several reflective essays and getting feedback from colleagues and senior staff. This is a preregistration requisite. Thankfully, in vet nursing CPD is still based on attendance only but in the future recording your post-CPD thought process may be required. This is not likely to be an in-depth process but understanding how reflection works will help make it a beneficial and less onerous task.

I was part of the RCVS trial group for outcome-based recording of CPD and during my time I wrote the following.

Reflection – rebranded

Oh, it is the R word again. Please do not turn off! I'm thinking we need to rebrand reflection as the word seems to cause such negativity in people. It is really just a process of reviewing new information and applying it to your life. So, could we just go for R&A?

The reason I am considering this is that I am doing some R&A for myself. Partly because I am now going through my BSAVA notes and partly because I am part of the RCVS pilot scheme for outcome-based CPD. I have wanted to improve how I record my CPD via the Professional Development Record (PDR) for a while. I have felt that what I record does not fully show what I have learned and what I have thought about it.

The pilot scheme introduction day at the RCVS earlier this year was really good. Informative and a great chance to talk to others with lots of different viewpoints. It felt that whatever comes out of this the college will get a range of views from across the industry, which was the intention.

My R&A from the pilot day was to consider asking some questions about any CPD I attend:

- What have you learnt?
- What will you do differently?

This can be done in easy bullet points – I will show you my efforts from a BSAVA lecture at the end. If you want to go a bit further you can consider expanding your thoughts:

- create headings to make your notes easy to review
- did the CPD relate to your objectives/thoughts at the start of the session or course?

There was some debate over the cycle of – plan, do, record, reflect – with some people having an issue over the planning stage. We know that we might head to a conference or congress and drop into a talk we had not planned on attending, or an evening CPD comes up that sounds interesting at short notice. We do not need to get stuck on the planning, it can be as simple as 'that sounds interesting' and going to an event. Or it can be a longer-term plan to learn new surgical techniques or undertake a post-graduation qualification. Both are equal in their planning – if you think you could learn something then do it.

I have found with teaching students R&A that there does come a point where you have to make sure it is a positive experience. The process should not become one where you are negative about yourself, and this includes deciding when to stop with the reflective cycle. May (2017) provides some great guidance on this:

- specific needs are met – for that individual patient/assessment
- general needs are met – for your overall body of knowledge/skills.

For some clinical cases it was also correctly suggested to consider: Is it worth starting . . . does the patient need a referral?

Finally, when is your new learning enough – when you are confident you can resolve the challenge? Yes, you could go and learn more but resolve the issue you have first.

I promised I'd give you my version of R&A for some BSAVA lectures so here is how I approach making notes in CPD lectures. . .

I have put together my list of questions and information to include on my PDR – in fact I have suggested that we can have a document on the PDR where you can store your R&A prompts to copy and paste onto the comments section, making life a little easier.

For each lecture, I made notes as I listened, as I always do. It would also be nice to upload those onto the PDR and use it as a one stop shop for notes. Now I've read back on my notes I have considered:

- new information
- changes to current working practice
- future plans.

I attended a lecture on alternative pain therapies. Something close to my heart for myself and for my elderly Persian Little Blue (LB). The lecture covered a number of alternative therapies and the results of research into their efficacy.

Here are my R&A notes on alternative pain therapies.

New info

- Acupuncture appears most effective (studies on dogs).
- Laser therapy is effective, but few negative studies so is there an issue with data?
- TENS machines effective but only for short term use, but can get owners to use at home.

Changes

- Consider TENS machine use in practice and for clients.

Future plans

- More info on laser and TENS machines, nurse led clinics for pain.

Yes, there was a lot more information provided in this lecture, and I am sure someone else's review of the lecture would be different. But that is the point of reflection. It is individual to the person and the practice, and it does not have to be a laborious process. Writing the blog and reviewing my notes has taken less than 1 hour. I will spend a little more time editing this as it's for publication but if it was not, I would leave it here and head to the PDR and copy and paste my notes in. It is that simple. Do not let the R word put you off. Call it what you like but do it!

You may find that as a result of reviewing CPD events and notes that you start writing a little more, which is never a bad thing. Writing is a good way of expressing yourself and if writing is not for you then most smart phones have audio note-making software. Or you can download an app that allows you to make audio notes that either allow you to play back the audio or turn them into written notes.

However you do it, you may well start to consider sharing what you have created. You may be asked to write for your employer in a number of different capacities so I have some ideas and tips for doing that next.

Writing

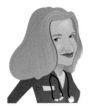

I'll start by saying – please don't be scared of writing.

It is not like writing as a task at school or for a grade at college. For many writing needs post qualification you are writing for your personal or practice needs and that allows some more freedom in what you produce than when writing for academic assessment. Publications will have guidelines for you and I have

'Words are, in my not-so-humble opinion, our most inexhaustible source of magic. Capable of both inflicting injury, and remedying it.'
– J.K. Rowling, Harry Potter and the Deathly Hallows

found great support from journals and companies alike so please do not be afraid to approach people and places with an idea of what you want to write.

Writing for publication

I cannot express enough how much we need vet nursing writing and research published. Whether that is in peer-reviewed journals or well-structured blogs, the vet nurse voice needs to be heard and there are many different mediums to write for. It might help to produce some informal pieces for your practice's Facebook page or the website to see how you find the experience and get some feedback from colleagues. Practices often need content for their social media and website so do offer some ideas you would like to write about.

Writing for publication does require some standards even if it is for your own blog. Head to Chapters Two and Three for advice on spelling, grammar and punctuation, and other basics.

Writing for journals

This can seem to be a most intimidating type of writing, as scientific writing is a very structured format and you need to be able to research your ideas as well as formulate them with the evidence you have found. You will need to spend more time on this type of writing than the other options and your initial idea and thoughts on the subject may well change when you start finding out more information. It is this aspect that can make peer-reviewed journal writing more interesting than just blogging about your favourite things.

Before publication you will most likely receive feedback on all aspects of the article and you will likely need to make changes. It is rare that anyone produces a new article and submits it and it gets published with no changes at all. Please do not be put off by this – it is *not* a sign that your work is not good enough. It is the process that all journal articles go through and it will make the writing easier each time you do it. It also helps spot the easy to miss typos and spelling mistakes that are hard to see when you have been reading your own work.

You will also need to have an understanding of Harvard referencing so head to Chapter Three to see how this works.

Blogging

This can be a nice way to explore if writing is for you. Start by exploring a few topics and carrying out some basic research. The blogs could be for your own use (not shared), your own blog that you do share, or for your employer or for many of the veterinary companies who need content created.

It is super easy to start your own website or set up on a blog hosting site. Some of these are free for basic features and include well-known names such as WordPress, or you can pay a fee for advanced features or a full website.

Blog is short for 'weblog' and it started as a way for people to use the web as a diary/journal. This meaning has changed slightly in that the posts do not have to follow the chronological course of your life. Blogs are usually informed opinion pieces of 300–900 words in length and as they are web based they allow for links to other information and products – called 'read throughs'. I like to use these as a way of evidencing what I have written and show how I came to the conclusions that I have. Think of it as an informal Harvard referencing.

However, do be clear on what is fact and opinion, do not fall into the trap of stating an opinion as fact. This is wrong, and can land you in a lot of trouble. Sharing your opinion is important but it also reflects on the whole profession so remain professional and adhere to the appropriate professional guidelines.

 A link to my articles on janervn.com is also available in the online resources.

Writing for speaking

Presenting your work as a lecture or workshop is a great way to share what you are passionate about. This could be to colleagues as part of a CPD sharing scheme at work, a presentation at a careers event or at a conference or congress.

Regardless of your audience, writing down what you want to say first is really important. There are ways to write to help you articulate what you say and create a speech or presentation without making it sound like you are reading from a script.

I have covered some of the ways to research and prepare for oral exams in Chapter Six and this will show you some ideas about writing for speaking. With presentations that are not for exams you have a lot of flexibility and, therefore, can focus on the subject and the audience and your own personal style.

Use the ideas of writing for an oral exam as a basis, and then add in your personal 'key points' and hook words that help the flow of your talk. Some words will help you with your timing and others as a key to memory.

By writing out a 'speech' in headings, and key words and phrases that you need to mention under that heading you can avoid the scripted feel of some presentations and also give yourself space to tailor the tone to the audience, the setting and the response you are getting. It is also a lot easier to remember and also much nicer for attendees if they see you with small notes and not pages of size 10 font typed notes to read from!

Flashcards can be helpful here too and you can put a timed amount of information on each card, which will help with timing and pacing. Where you would have a paragraph in an essay or blog you can have a flash card with notes to prompt you.

Figure 9.2 shows examples of layout options for presentations that you can fill in with the information from your research. They remind you of the structure of the talk and break it down into small segments and give timings and which slides from a presentation will be shown at that part of your talk.

Where you have research to share, you can display this on your visual presentation, which can be an electronic presentation, or a pre-prepared poster– it really depends on the subject and the audience.

I have found when presenting anatomy sessions that drawing – however basically – as you go along is a better educational tool than presenting beautiful images or drawings. However, for other subjects, for example anaesthesia then presenting graphs and professional images and statistics would be expected. Any visual aid needs to be acknowledged in your written notes so you do not forget to link your talking and your visual information – as per the flashcard guides above.

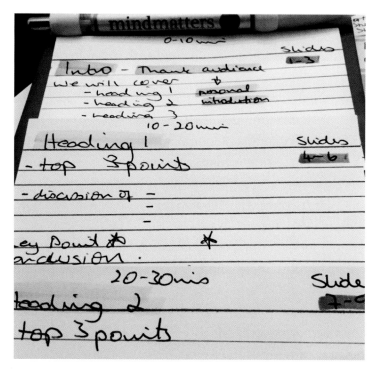

Figure 9.2 Example of note making format for public speaking

Despite all the best laid plans presentations do not always go as you planned. The joy of a talk is that your audience does not have your notes and so will most likely not know if you have deviated from them or changed the order of the key points.

This is also a good time to say that you can create a visual presentation and *not* be a slave to PowerPoint or Key Note – they should augment and support your presentation. You usually find less is more with text on visual presentations so keep the writing on them brief and focus on diagrams, pictures and graphs.

Knowledge summary and PICO – evidence-based veterinary medicine

You may wish to join with the evidence-based veterinary medicine groups and work to create a **knowledge summary** of a subject area you are interested in. A knowledge summary is similar to a literature review but your search areas and presentation of data are restricted. This means they focus on the facts and you are not forming an opinion as you would if writing a literature review essay. It also means they are quicker to produce than an essay and the format is accessible to all.

A knowledge summary starts with a question formed with the help of PICO:

Patient/population	–	who is affected?
Intervention	–	what is the treatment?
Comparisons	–	what can this be compared to?
Outcomes	–	what happens to the patients? (Northedge, 2005)

We are again back to our Kipling friends: who, what, when, where, why and how.

A rough idea for building a PICO is as follows.

Creating a question from your experience can help focus what it is you wish to find out more about. Background information from your description should start with:

1. a question route with a verb: does, can, etc.
2. an aspect of the condition or thing of interested – B12 in cats.

Then make a simple question such as – In cats with renal failure is B12 of benefit?

You will then foreground questions that ask for specific knowledge to inform clinical decision or actions. You can add much more information with this type of questioning and this structures your research and the papers you will find. As chronic renal failure (CRF) in older cats is a relatively common disease there will be a lot of research on this and not all of it will be relevant to your search. It can be easy to get into an information overload if you start searching before you have narrowed down your search.

A simple attempt at a PICO involves:

Feline, geriatric, CRF	Patient, population, predicament or problem
B12	Intervention, exposure, test or other agent
Other supplements	Comparison intervention, exposure, test
Reducing trips to vets	Outcomes of clinical importance, including time when relevant

Final question to be answered:

In geriatric cats with CRF what regimes of B12 supplement are most beneficial with minimal visit to the vets?

You can do more with a PICO and expand it to a full table to increase the search term options. As an example, if you are interested in finding any information on treating diabetic cats with medication that does not require injections – as you have encountered many clients who do not like the concept of injecting their cat daily and do not feel able to do this – how do you find the information that gives helpful information?

The PICO table gives you the search terms you will use in your database and is useful even when not researching a knowledge summary. It can help you to break down the information you need for an SOP or when handling a case you wish to research further care for.

As Straus et al. (2010: 17) say:

Lifelong learning skills need to be built to practice EBM. To use knowledge wisely learners need hard work and coaching, concentrating on such things as reflection, to recognize their own learning needs.

To fully integrate evidence-based veterinary medicine you need to be asking clinical questions that are answerable. There is little point in searching for information that, while interesting, will not help your quest for knowledge or help you regularly with your patients.

Training others

As many RVNs know you will often be called upon to help train others. From receptionists' first days to final year vet students and everyone in between. While it is great that it is clear to others our skills set is varied and standards high, it can add to your workload.

There is information on coaching and mentoring in Appendix A – looking at the coaching process from the student's point of view. It covers common coaching models and how to work successfully as a coach. This can easily be applied to being the coach and while you may not need to use the models for all training situations they are a handy thing to know about and use when motivating staff with training.

Training others involves the art of delegation. It can be hard to have to step back from certain jobs we may have always done and hand them over to someone else. Training others can be a process in which you can learn to delegate and feel comfortable with doing so. To delegate properly you will need to consider how you recognize roles in practice and how your team works.

Coaching is classed as 'the facilitation of learning', where there is no set direction, unlike in mentoring. Employers can improve the performance and motivation of their staff through coaching. The coaching process looks to provide support, challenges, feedback and give guidance to employees' decision making, rather than to make decisions for them. Employees then feel able to use their awareness and the responsibility of their role to achieve the best they can. It has changed many workplaces and coaching is moving from being an individual process to a team process. The purpose remains the same, to allow employees to achieve their full potential. It should continuously lead to improvements in the capability and/or conduct of the employee and the team they are in.

Personal welfare

I started this book some months ago and in the first pages put some information about self-care and some helpful phone numbers. This is not to shock or scare anyone that life as a vet nurse or vet nurse student is so bad you will need these numbers from just reading this book, but rather taking a moment to say that by reading any type of book for help or support you may realize that some more help and support is needed. Something beyond the pages of a book. You can refer back to Chapter One for more info on this. There are people to help you, so please do not be alone and worry if you do not feel good.

As an RVN you may have the added pressure of training a veterinary nurse and supporting vet students during their training. Remember to take care of yourself too.

I could spout a thousand Facebook memes here but all you really need to know is that if a client came in and said their dog had not eaten or slept properly for 3 days and did not want to go for a walk then you would say that something is wrong and advise them to get help.

Treat yourself like you would a patient and get help. That help for you can come in any form you need it to take. Going to your favourite place, cooking a nice meal, seeing friends, even a nice hot bath. My personal preferences are:

- a sunset paddleboard
- Co-op sea salt and chardonnay wine vinegar crisps
- prosecco
- re-reading a familiar book, *Harry Potter, Northern Lights, The Great Gatsby*
- watching a familiar film – as with the books or *The Hunger Games, Dangerous Liaisons.*

But you can change this list!

Something to try to relax, unwind and reward yourself. If these short-term measures do not improve your feelings then please do consider talking to someone to try to work out what is wrong, and what can be done about it. You are not alone if you do not feel like the life and soul of the party 24/7 and you do not need to be, you just need to be you.

Review Chapter 9 and how to apply what you have learned with the Reflective Template.

> *'When gone am I, the last of the Jedi will you be. The Force runs strong in your family. Pass on what you have learned.'*
> — *Yoda*, Star Wars, Episode VI – Return of the Jedi

Chapter Nine glossary

Boolean search – a way to use search engines

continuing professional development – system of recording post qualification education

knowledge summary – an RCVS Knowledge system where literature reviews of subject areas are carried out and reported in an easily accessible manner

qualification – one leading to veterinary nurse status

RACE – registry approved continuing education, US system of CPD

The clinical coach/ supervisor

In the UK for every student there is a CC and as we want to increase the number of SVNs then we will need to see an increase in CCs too. Yes, you can have more than one SVN as a CC

You sign up as a training 'practice' not as a training 'person'.

but it is better to spread the workload. In other schemes, you will find clinical supervisors, mentors and other student support roles.

I feel it is very important to say that not all RVNs or member of the Royal College of Veterinary Surgeons (MRCVS) want to be a CC. That is fine, forcing people to take on this role rarely goes well. But you could sell the idea to people.

What do you gain from being a CC?

Being a CC can help you improve your own skills. You need to be organized and plan your and the student's time. It can be another great avenue for CPD, a move from a clinical focus to coaching and mentoring skills. You learn so much about yourself when doing this type of work it is of great benefit to you personally and the team.

There is nothing like someone asking questions about your clinical skills to make you improve your own skills. What is the latest on skin prep for surgery? Does your SOP for kennel cleaning have an evidence base? It is a great reason to use the student's access to knowledge and training to review your practices and make sure you are happy with your patient care.

The R word is an important consideration for all of us. Reflection can be hard for some people but you will be glad to hear that there is evidence that those who supervise others find their skills and reflection are improved. You work with the student to aid their reflection and this helps your own.

Clients also adore the fact they are with a practice that trains students. They love to hear about the training process and the care taken of their pets. They understand that training means there is supervision and this is good for patient care. Lately I have seen more practices announcing students qualifying on their practice social media – a great marketing tool if you want to be cynical – but also a great way to celebrate the team that created the basis for success.

What do you do?

You're coming round to the idea? Possibly? What do you actually do? I will add my twist to the way Ali Heywood – course director at College of West Anglia – describes it, I think of it as the 3Ps.

Pragmatic

- Being sensible and reasonable and honest about the SVNs practical skills.

Practical

- Being able to spend time with the SVN on their practical skills.
- Having the skills to work with clinical skill as from start of training to Day One skills.

Pom-poms

- Ali says be your student's cheerleader – I think of waving pom-poms.
- Including them in the team.
- Ensuring their needs are included in team plans.

With the benefits you get, is it that much of a task? Come on, join in.

> 'Most people never get to see how brilliant they can be. They don't find teachers that believe in them. They get convinced they're stupid.'
> – Sean Maguire, Good Will Hunting

WBL records

Like many people I qualified with the National Vocational Qualifications (NVQ) portfolio. It was such a behemoth of a file, physically and emotionally, and by the time it was finished. It was so precious I moved house with it three times.

> *Finally, I accepted I had my RVN qualification and that the RCVS would not come knocking to read it.*

I checked for any sensitive information and put it in recycling, quite a momentous day.

I liked some aspects of the portfolio, but really love being a CC for the NPL. It is focused on your practical skills, not how well you write about them. My only negative has been that the breakdown of it into tasks makes the students forget about logging the experience of nursing the whole patient – they can get set on their list of tasks to complete. I have found this means they can miss the importance of everyday skills while they focus on the individual 'exciting' or hard to find ones. Comparing this to the portfolio where we wrote about nursing the patient for extended periods it can make a student's move towards becoming a proficient practitioner a little more stilted.

But nothing stays the same in education as it changes to stay abreast of changes in the industry. I am pleased to say there are some great changes to the NPL, reflecting a move towards encouraging students to look at the experience they gain from the whole patient.

The updated NPL has fewer individual tasks and fewer sections – the tasks are now together in ten sections. The tasks are being linked now not through the unit but by the way we would do them when faced with a patient. Placing the focus back on the skill of nursing and not just the small individual tasks that make this up. This will encourage the students to log their experience of being with a patient for an extended period of time, not just cherry picking the skills they need.

While this will mean a period of adjustment for current CCs it will streamline the NPL. The repetition of skills across more than one unit is reduced. Meaning if you have logged a great wound in one area you do not then open another to find you could have used it there too. It also focuses the student on gaining as much from one patient as possible. Which is great for quieter practices. I have encountered some students who were concerned they do not see enough patients as they worried about logging too many tasks on one patient.

The updated NPL also includes a behaviour section. Not for the patient's behaviour but for the student's. If you have had degree students you will be familiar with their behavioural tool. A way to grade the student's attitude and aptitude while on placement. The new NPL requires input at various points in the student's progress. This is taken from the several sources providing a view of the students conduct outside of purely academic progress. While students are not under the jurisdiction of the disciplinary committee while studying we need to ensure that they understand what good, professional conduct is and what is not acceptable for when they qualify. This behavioural section provides a structure for issues to be raised and hopefully resolved. It is not there to prevent people qualifying but to support people through a tough training process and create well rounded professionals.

It all adds up to a holistic nursing education producing well rounded professionals. A step in the right direction.

Student contract

One aspect of training and supporting staff that is rarely set out by the practice is the conduct expected. I have found many practices that rely on the college student contract for enforcing behaviour, or attendance at both college and practice. Before the student enters into their course they should know what the practice expects of them. They have a set number of hours to achieve in practice to be able to qualify, they have behavioural assessments by college tutors and colleagues at work. This goes above and beyond employment law and are guidelines you can use in practice. As a tutor, I often heard views of what seemed like two very different people when asking about behaviour in college and at work. If students know there are the same standards in both places then they are more likely to adhere to them and there is less likely to be an issue where they play college off against practice. It also helps the student understand the boundaries of their role and the best way to progress to academic and professional success.

> *Linked in with behaviour and attendance is achievement.*

It is surprising to me how many practices have nothing in their contract about when they expect the student to achieve and what happens if they do not achieve by that deadline. If there is a business plan to have more RVNs and training them is the way to achieve this you need to know when the transition from SVN to RVN will occur.

It affects the team structure, future recruitment plans and rota. Most courses are 2 or 3 years for a diploma student. What happens if a student has not achieved consistently well to qualify in that time period? Yes, they are able to continue and can complete the course at a slower rate, in the time scale given to achieve a course. But how does that impact on the employer? Are you able to support a student for that long? Do you need to review your recruitment plans and team structure, if you now do not have the RVN you thought you would have.

These are things most student nurses do not consider when they start. They think the practice will always have space to accommodate them and they can achieve at their own pace. While this is true in many cases, funding a student through vet nurse training is a cost to the business and ongoing support needs to be justified if the positives of gaining an RVN is not going to happen when originally planned.

This then raises the issue of how the employer deals with ongoing achievement and how employer and employee communicate. Is there contact with the college during term rather than waiting for end of term reports? Are all parties aware of test results and assignment marks? If there are any resits needed and when these are for, it is prudent to know these things to ensure both parties are getting the best from the training process and that they are keeping to the contract on achievement.

Having employment as an RVN after training is complete and undertaking new responsibilities once qualified should both be discussed before starting training. If there is a contractual obligation to remain with the practice post-qualification for a certain period there is a need to check with employment specialists about exactly how long this can be for – as part of supporting someone through their training, financially and practically – it is accepted that they give back to the practice during and once training is complete. This can be as a qualified member of staff ensuring you have an RVN for a set period of time and it may also mean undertaking more responsibilities.

> *For success both the student and the practice need a clear contract of obligations and expectations, making for a more beneficial partnership.*

Creative teaching and learning opportunities

While we can be creative as students, lecturers, tutors and clinical coaches may also need some ideas to promote creativity in learning. During my time teaching I have developed some educational tools based on popular quizzes and games, adding familiarity to new subject areas and an opportunity to relax and learn.

Vet nurse dictionary Pictionary

The popular drawing game requires players to communicate a word via their own drawing of it. The 'real rules' involve a board game and playing in teams but I have simplified it by not using a board and not always opting to move a class into teams.

Timing is optional! The 'dictionary' can be of your choice but obviously try and use texts from your course reading list. Some topics and words lend themselves better to this format than others and its really successful for anatomy and physiology.

Imaging Blockbusters

Blockbusters is a game that ages you! Yes, I am old enough to remember watching it on TV and sniggering at people asking 'can I have a Pee please Bob' – it was before we had the internet so we can be excused.

The aim of the game is to answer question correctly to claim coloured blocks on the board to link from left to right, or top to bottom. A team of two people works across the board, which is the longer route, and a single player works top to bottom, the shorter route.

The blocks all contain a single letter and it is the first letter of the correct answer, so that's pretty easy? The questions are all phrased the same and lend themselves to practising multiple choice questions. For example, they might ask:

'What E can cause a yellowing of a radiographic image over time?'
Answer – exhausted fixer.

This style of questioning is easy to replicate in many subject areas and templates for a blank board are available online for free, try searching 'blank blockbusters board'.

I have created great games for imaging and for exotics too. You just need a broad enough subject area that means you can get three or four questions per letter of the alphabet.

Vet nurse dictionary corner

Dictionary corner is good for subjects that do not lend themselves to visual representation or to simple answers such as in Blockbusters.

Getting students to come up with their own definitions of words can be a great way to learn and also to share and compare their definitions.

These sessions can be set as students presenting to the class or as a small group swap and discuss session.

Dragons' Den

A popular way to engage a class is to have students research and 'pitch' an idea to a panel just as in *Dragons' Den*. The style of presenting means students are evaluating their given area, which is a great skill to have. Critiquing different options for patient skin prep prior to surgery or is washing and re-sterilising cloth drapes better than disposable?

The subjects to debate are endless and the creativity in students is unlimited!

Bibliography

Adams, R., Fowler, M. and Lomis, K. (2003) Enhancing clinical skills coaching via a cohort of faculty trained and supported to conduct direct observations in the workplace. Available at: https://medschool.vanderbilt.edu/mctp/files/mctp/public_files/MCTabstractforAAMC.pdf (accessed 20 May 2018).

Apsinall, V. (2006) *The Complete Textbook of Veterinary Nursing.* Elsevier, London.

Baillie, S. and Rhind, S. (2008) A guide to assessment methods in veterinary medicine. Available at: http://www.live.ac.uk/Media/LIVE/PDFs/assessment_guide.pdf (accessed 14 May 2017).

Benjamin, L., Cavell, T.A. and Shallenberger, III, W.R. (1984) Staying with initial answers on objective tests: is it a myth? *Teaching of Psychology* 11(3), 133–141.

Boyd, C. (2014) *Study Skills for Nurses.* Wiley and Sons, Chichester.

Bradford University (2014) E-advice - grammar, spelling and punctuation analysis. Available at: http://www.brad.ac.uk/academic-skills/media/academics killsadvice/documents/exemplars/WHAT-TO-EXPECT-FROM-E-ADVICE---GRAMMAR-ANALYSIS.pdf (accessed 4 March 2017).

BSAVA (n.d.) https://www.bsava.com/Resources/Veterinary-resources/Medicines-Guide/Storage-and-dispensary-management (accessed 19 September 2018).

CABi (n.d.) https://www.cabi.org/ (accessed 12 February 2017).

Cascrini, L. (2004) Surviving a viva: a guide for candidates. Available at: https://www.ncbi.nlm.nih.gov/pmc/articles/PMC1079624/ (accessed 14 May 2017).

CASP (2014) Critical appraisal skills programme. Available at: http://www.casp-uk.net/ (accessed 15 February 2017).

Center for the Enhancement of Learning & Teaching (n.d.) One minute paper. Available at: http://provost.tufts.edu/celt/files/MinutePaper.pdf (accessed 14 December 2016).

City and Guilds (2015) 7457 Veterinary Nurse Reading List. Available at: https://cdn.cityandguilds.com/ProductDocuments/Land_Based_Services/Animal_

Management/7457/7457_Level_3/Centre_documents/7457_Veterinary_
Nursing_Reading_List_v3.pdf (accessed 21 February 2018).

City and Guilds (2017) Level 3 Diploma sample paper. Available only to
registered users.

Costandi, M. (2016) If you can't imagine things, how can you learn? *Guardian*
4 June. Available at: https://www.theguardian.com/education/2016/jun/04/
aphantasia-no-visual-imagination-impact-learning (accessed 11 April 2017).

Cottrell, S. (2013) *The Study Skills Handbook.* 4th edn. Palgrave McMillan,
London.

CVTEA Accreditation Policies and Procedures - Appendix I (2018) Essential and
recommended skills for vet tech students. Available at: https://www.avma.
org/ProfessionalDevelopment/Education/Accreditation/Programs/Pages/
cvtea-pp-appendix-i.aspx (accessed 12 February 2018).

Cybertext (2012) A light-hearted look at how punctuation can change meaning.
Available at: https://cybertext.wordpress.com/2012/11/22/a-light-hearted-
look-at-how-punctuation-can-change-meaning/ (accessed 7 March 2017).

Davidson, J. (2016) Jane RVN. Available at: https://www.youtube.com/channel/
UCAnLRvAfHVTxuHvokzkTPlw (accessed 13 April 2017).

Davidson, J. (2017) Veterinary nursing uniforms: their role in infection control.
The Veterinary Nurse 8(1), 6–10.

De Montfort University (2013) How to undertake a literature search and review
for dissertations and final year projects. Available at: http://www.library.
dmu.ac.uk/Images/Howto/LiteratureSearch.pdf (accessed 3 March 2017).

Dreyfus, S.E. (2004) The five-stage model of adult skill acquisition. *Bulletin of
Science Technology & Society* 24, 177.

Du. M. (2017) RCVS Knowledge. Available at: http://knowledge.rcvs.org.uk/
home/ (accessed 15 February 2017).

Dunn, L.S. (n.d.) Standard operating procedures for your animal hospital.
Available at: https://www.veterinaryteambrief.com/sites/default/files/
Standard-Operating-Procedures.pdf (accessed 6 June 2017).

Graduate School (n.d.) Practice viva questions. Available at: http://www2.le.ac.
uk/departments/gradschool/training/eresources/study-guides/viva/prepare/
questions (accessed 14 May 2017).

Ilkiw, J.E. (2017) Integrated learning. In: Hodgson, J.L. and Pelzer, J.M. (eds)
Veterinary Medical Education. A Practical Guide. Wiley Blackwell, Chichester,
pp. 66–68.

Jasper, M. (2003) *Beginning Reflective Practice*. Nelson Thornes, Cheltenham.

Jetstream Publishing Limited (n.d.) Veterinary nurse training – examples. Available at: http://www.veterinary-nursing.co.uk/examples/mcq.htm (accessed 3 April 2017).

Jstor (n.d.) Available at: https://www.jstor.org/ (accessed 5 February 2017).

Kelly, M., Lyng, C., McGrath, M. and Cannon, G. (2009) A multi-method study to determine the effectiveness of, and student attitudes to, online instructional videos for teaching clinical nursing skills. *Nurse Education Today* 29(3), 292–300.

Kennedy, C. (n.d.) Update on peer assisted learning. Available at: https://www.amee.org/getattachment/AMEE-Initiatives/MedEdWorld/38074-Peer-Assisted-Learning-WEB.PDF (accessed 21 May 2017).

Laerd (2012a) STAGE 1 - Getting to the main journal article. Available at: http://dissertation.laerd.com/process-stage1.php (accessed 3 March 2017).

Laerd (2012b) Statistics in your dissertation. Available at: https://statistics.laerd.com/ (accessed 3 March 2017).

Magnier, K. and Paed, M. (2017) Performance and workplace-based assessment. In: Hodgson, J.L. and Pelzer, J.M. (eds) *Veterinary Medical Education: A Practical Guide*. Wiley and Sons, Chichester, pp. 255–272.

May, S. (2017) Reflection and our professional lives. *Livestock* 22(1), 33–37.

Media First (n.d.) Available at: https://www.mediafirst.co.uk/our-thinking/vibrant-varied-and-still-going-strong-a-guide-to-uk-newspaper-audiences/ (accessed 14 November 2018).

Moore, M. and Palmer, N. (2001) *Calculations for Veterinary Nurses*. Blackwells, Oxford.

Muralitharan, N. and Peate, I. (2001) Fundamentals of anatomy and physiology for nursing and healthcare students. Available at: http://www.fundamentalsofanatomy.com/mcqs/mcq.asp?I=1444334433&chapter=09&q=0010 (accessed 3 April 2017).

NHS (2018) Breathing for stress. Available at: http://www.nhs.uk/conditions/stress-anxiety-depression/pages/ways-relieve-stress.aspx (accessed 14 December 2016).

F. Nind and P. Mosedale (eds) (2018) *BSAVA Guide to the Use of Veterinary Medicines*. BSAVA, Quedgeley.

Northedge, A. (2005) *The Good Study Guide*. Open Univeristy Press, Milton Keynes.

PESTLEanalysis Contributor (2013) SWOT analysis examples for every business situation. Available at: http://pestleanalysis.com/swot-analysis-examples/ (accessed 21 May 2017).

Pubmed (n.d.) Available at: https://www.ncbi.nlm.nih.gov/pubmed/ (accessed 5 February 2017).

RCVS (2002) Advice and guidance. Available at: http://www.rcvs.org.uk/advice-and-guidance/code-of-professional-conduct-for-veterinary-surgeons/supporting-guidance/delegation-to-veterinary-nurses/ (accessed 1 December 2016).

RCVS (2015) Code of conduct. Available at: http://www.rcvs.org.uk/advice-and-guidance/code-of-professional-conduct-for-veterinary-nurses/supporting-guidance/delegation-to-veterinary-nurses/ (accessed 5 December 2016).

Rennie, I. (2009) Exploring approaches to clinical skills development in nursing education. *Nursing Times* 105(3), 20–22.

Skillworks Toolkit (2013) Coaching for college and career. Available at: http://www.skill-works.org/documents/SkillWorksCoachingToolkit_WebOnly.pdf (accessed 21 May 2017).

Solent Online Learning (2017) Kolb's learning cycle. Available at: http://learn.solent.ac.uk/mod/book/view.php?id=2732&chapterid=1112 (accessed 14 December 2016).

Sparky Teaching (2014) Blog - mean, median, mode and range. Available at: http://www.sparkyteaching.com/creative/free-averages-poster/ (accessed 11 April 2017).

Straus, S., Glasziou, W.P., Scott Richardson, R. and Haynes, B. (2010) *Evidence Based Medicine and How to Practice and Teach*. 4th edn. Churchill Livingstone, London.

Teekman, B. (2000) Exploring reflective thinking in nursing practice. *Journal of Advanced Nursing* 31, 1125–1135.

Thomas, J.T.N. (2014) Ancient imagery mnemonics. Available at: https://plato.stanford.edu/entries/mental-imagery/ancient-imagery-mnemonics.html (accessed 11 April 2017).

Truss, L. (2009) *Eats, Shoots and Leaves*. Harper Collins, London.

Unit for the Enhancement of Learning and Teaching (2013) Viva voce exams for taught undergraduate and postgraduate programmes. Available at: https://www.kent.ac.uk/teaching/qa/guidance/viva.html (accessed 17 May 2017).

University College Los Angeles (2017) Phrases versus keyword searching. Available at: http://guides.library.ucla.edu/databases/techniques#s-lg-box-3596165 (accessed 15 February 2017).

University of Kent (2008) Instruction verbs in essay questions. Available at: https://www.kent.ac.uk/ai/ask/documents/step_1_Instruction_verbs.pdf (accessed 3 April 2017).

University of Southampton (n.d.) Memory, revision and exam techniques. Available at: https://www.southampton.ac.uk/assets/imported/transforms/content-block/UsefulDownloads_Download/3F82D0A1F6F34D62AC4D DBFF3A4BAFDE/Memory%20revision%20and%20exam%20techniques% 202014.pdf (accessed 1 December 2016).

University of Toronto (n.d.) http://www.utoronto.ca/writing/litrev.html (accessed 13 November 2018).

University of Waterloo (n.d.) Exam questions: types, characteristics and suggestions. Available at: https://uwaterloo.ca/centre-for-teaching-excellence/teaching-resources/teaching-tips/developing-assignments/exams/questions-types-characteristics-suggestions (accessed 11 April 2017).

Veterinary Nurses Council of Australia (n.d.) Code of conduct for veterinary nurses. Available at: http://www.vnca.asn.au/public/11/files/Membership/CODE-OF-CONDUCT_web.pdf (accessed 12 February 2018).

Wass, V., Wakeford, R., Neighbour, R. and Van der Vleuten C. (2003) Achieving acceptable reliability in oral examinations: an analysis of the Royal College of General Practitioners membership examination's oral component. *Medical Education* 37(2), 126–131.

Yale University (n.d.) The web vs. library databases – a comparison. Available at: https://www.library.yale.edu/researcheducation/pdfs/Searching_Evaluating_Resources.pdf (accessed 22 February 2017).